Risky Sex

Between Men ~

Between Women

Lesbian and Gay Studies

Lillian Faderman and Larry Gross, Editors

Risky Sex

Gay Men and HIV Prevention

Dwayne C. Turner

Columbia University Press

New York

Columbia University Press
Publishers Since 1893
New York   Chichester, West Sussex

Library of Congress Cataloging-in-Publication Data
Turner, Dwayne Curtis
    Risky sex : gay men and HIV prevention / Dwayne C. Turner.
    p.   cm. — (Between men—between women)
    Includes bibliographical references and index.
    ISBN 0–231–10574-6 (alk. paper). — ISBN 0–231–10575–4 (pbk. :
alk. paper)
    1. Gay men—California—West Hollywood—Sexual behavior. 2. Safe
sex in AIDS prevention—California—West Hollywood.   I. Title.
II. Series.
HQ76.2.U52W477   1997
306.7'086'642—dc21   96–40290

Casebound editions of Columbia University Press books are
printed on permanent and durable acid-free paper.

Printed in the United States of America

c 10 9 8 7 6 5 4 3 2 1
p 10 9 8 7 6 5 4 3 2 1

Contents

Acknowledgments

Many people contributed either directly or indirectly to the final outcome of this book. Some were my teachers. Some are my friends. Others listened to my thoughts and/or reviewed versions of this manuscript. Others may have helped without even knowing it. After all is written and done, I appreciate the generous help, support, and encouragement from the following individuals and organizations: AIDS Project Los Angeles, Robert Bailey, Christy Beaudin, Ralph Bolton, Robert Boyd and Joan Silk (for opening my mind), Lindsay Braverman (for his love), Francesca Bray, William Cunningham, Jennifer Furin, Douglas Hollan, Inez Holley (Mom), Jessie, Lee Klosinski, Cathy Martin, Marty and Stephan (the Other Two Heathers), Anil Mohin (he knows why), Donald Morisky (and all the students, myself included, who were fortunate enough to participate in his AIDS training grant at UCLA), Jon Olson, Nadine Peacock, Deborah Riopelle, Eve Rubell, Karen Sacks, Kirsten Senturia, Amy Tauber, Ann Walters (graduate advisor extraordinaire), and Timothy Welch.

Particular appreciation must go to the State of California University-wide AIDS Research Program for its financial support, Susan C. M. Scrimshaw for her guidance, Ann Miller at Columbia University Press for giving me this opportunity, and to all the courageous men who participated in this project.

Introduction: Embracing the Jaguar

Several friends have told me . . . that meeting a jaguar can change one's way of looking at the world.

—Murray Gell-Mann, *The Quark and the Jaguar* (1994)

They went out of that courtyard into another doorway, and up a great flight of steps and through vast rooms that opened out of one another till you were dizzy with the mere size of the place. Every now and then they thought they were going to get out into the open. . . . But each time they only got into another courtyard.

—C. S. Lewis, *The Magician's Nephew* (1955)

When I first entered graduate school in the fall of 1989, I planned to do a research project about homosexuality in Nicaragua. At that time, I had a Marxist bent and was curious about how the Sandinista government viewed homosexuality, both from a cultural and a political perspective. However, perhaps not unexpectedly, my plans changed direction as various twists and turns—in short, the vagaries of life—led me to conclude that I had work to do at home in Los Angeles, California.

One of the great and cruel events of the last decades of the twentieth century, Acquired Immune Deficiency Syndrome (AIDS), had struck and was wiping out a whole generation of young men, many of whom were my friends and acquaintances. Shortly after the Human Immunodeficiency Virus (HIV) antibody screening test became available, I took it and tested negative, but I was still horrified, frightened, and angry. With a zealous drive, I became involved with the political activist group ACT UP (AIDS Coalition to Unleash Power) in Los Angeles. In those years, ACT UP Los Angeles was a "grassroots, democratic, militant, direct action organization dedicated to creating positive changes around AIDS in federal and local government, the media, and the medical and pharmaceutical industries through non-violent public protests" (Turner 1991).

As a national movement, ACT UP sought access to medical treatments and lobbied the Food and Drug Administration (FDA) to speed up its drug approval process. The dedicated men and women of ACT UP achieved both these goals, while at the same time struggling to ease the discriminatory atmosphere manifest in governmental attitudes and legislation. Not everyone, whether gay or straight, approved of ACT UP's singularly styled, often confrontational, political tactics (camp juxtaposed with anger), but the group did accomplish much that it had set out to do.

In the epidemic's early years, activists were adamant that a cure could be found if the government and private industry would just get off their duffs, allocate more resources, and move at a more urgent and rapid pace. New drugs such as Zidovudine (better known as AZT), once tested and approved, showed some promise in slowing the disease process; meanwhile, endless gossip concerning new alternative and experimental treatments buzzed through meeting halls and AIDS agencies. Some people with HIV and their friends, taking research into their own hands in a race against time, even set up illegal medical laboratories in homes and basements.

In 1992 and 1993 the gossip took a pessimistic turn as hopes for an immediate cure dwindled and data from the Concorde trial (a huge clinical trial of antiretrovirals) were presented at the Ninth Annual International Conference on AIDS, held in Berlin (1993). The large Concorde study had involved seventy-three medical centers in cities throughout the United Kingdom, Ireland, and France and compared individuals receiving early treatment of the disease with AZT to those receiving a placebo. The results were disheartening. AZT appeared not to be the "magic bullet" that some had hoped and prayed it would be (Seligmann 1993). Indeed, after hearing the data from the Concorde trial, activists attending the conference fell into a sullen, almost resigned, mood.

For some, particularly HIV-infected activists, reality hit hard, and for others such as myself, our friends continued to die. Even before the Concorde trial data became known, however, some medical providers had already come to the unwelcome realization that the best they could hope for in present circumstances would be to "manage" HIV disease while the desperate search for a cure went on. Nevertheless, that summer in Berlin, both activists and researchers felt exhausted; still, they continued to work, sometimes together and sometimes in opposition.

At that same conference—at a plenary session entitled "Prevention: Is it Working?"—participants expressed doubts over how well education and prevention were succeeding in slowing the epidemic down (Lamptey et al. 1993). On the whole, the conference proved to be both a symbolic and real turning point in reflecting upon and evaluating treatment and prevention efforts to date. It was also a pivotal and sobering event for me, and I became somewhat less involved with treatment activism and turned my primary (though far from exclusive) focus to prevention education and behavioral research. For the first time, I came to know the true power of HIV, every gay man's jaguar.

The Berlin conference, indeed, spurred much of the philosophical direction of this book. Those of us attending that conference were, I believe, asking the wrong questions about HIV prevention. Rather than "Is it working?" we should be asking, "How effective have prevention efforts been and what can we do to make them better?" This latter question implicitly acknowledges the fact that there is currently no magic bullet either in treating AIDS or for changing sexual and drug use behaviors but, at the same time, it posits behavior change as an ongoing process and not just as an endpoint. Because these behaviors, both engaging in sex and the use of drugs, are considered by the individual to be pleasurable (that is, pleasurable vis-à-vis their cultural meanings as well as in any evolved physiological responses), their indulgence is not easily relinquished.

Seeing prevention as an ongoing process is to step back from all-or-nothing categories such as "working"/"not working" and to look at behavior change as a lifelong endeavor that involves making ambivalent decisions. These decisions blur discrete categories (such as "yes I will wear a condom" or "no I will not wear a condom") and are dependent upon time and space. Next week, for example, a gay man may intend to use a condom while having sex but then may penetrate his partner without one—at least initially, pulling out once he realizes what he is doing. A year from now, in a different time, a different setting, and with a different partner, he may use a condom during part of the sexual encounter or he may use it for the entire encounter—or it is possible that he may not use one at all. The variations are many, the possibilities endless.

Given the somewhat unpredictable (and, at the same time, somewhat predictable) elements of sexual encounters, all-or-nothing measures of the effectiveness of prevention programs, including measures like inconsistent and consistent use of condoms, set these programs, their participants, and educators up for failure. In short, binary categories do not and cannot tell us how well education and prevention are doing.

Instead of using binary-based logic, in this book I take a less restricted approach to illustrate and discern the blurred areas between binary extremes. Bart Kosko, in his book *Fuzzy Thinking: The New Science of Fuzzy Logic*, uses a familiar object, an apple, to demonstrate how limited these binary categories can be in describing change and how they do not allow for different settings and different times. He writes:

> Hold an apple in your hand. Is it an apple? Yes. The object in your hand belongs to the clumps of space-time we call the set of apples. . . . Now take a bite, chew it, swallow it. Let your digestive tract take apart the apple's molecules. Is the object in your hand still an apple? Yes or no? Take another bite. Is the new object still an apple? Take another bite and so on down to void. The apple changes from thing to nonthing to nothing. But where does it cross the line from apple to nonapple? When you hold half an apple in your hand, the apple is as much there as not. The half apple foils all-or-none descriptions. The half apple is a fuzzy apple, the gray between the black and the white. Fuzziness is grayness.
>
> (Kosko 1993:4)

By using fuzzy logic, I am not trying to make things more complicated. Nor am I attempting to appear overly erudite or esoteric. I am simply resisting a Western cultural tendency to see the world in black-and-white terms, a tendency traceable back to Aristotle.

Aristotle proposed three "laws" or rules to govern "logical" thought. Two of these laws are most relevant here as they are essential to all-or-nothing logic. The first of these, the "law" of noncontradiction, declares that a statement and its negation cannot be true at the same time. In the second law, the "law" of the excluded middle, Aristotle concluded that a statement cannot be both true and false (Coveney and Highfield 1995). In other words, using Aristotle's "laws," an apple cannot be a nonapple, there can be no "grain" of truth, and a person cannot somewhat agree or somewhat disagree with any given statement. He or she must simply agree or disagree. There is nothing in-between.

These laws of logic have been questioned by some mathematicians and applied scientists working in the area of technological development for their relevance to a real and fuzzy world in which phenomena rarely exist in black *or* white (Coveney and Highfield 1995; Kosko 1993; Zadeh 1965). "Our brains often reason with vague assertions, uncertainties, and value judgments," write Coveney and Highfield in regard to fuzzy logic. "Now there has been an attempt at constructing a logical model of human reasoning that reflects its approximate and qualitative nature" (1995). And Lotfi Zadeh, who wrote the landmark fuzzy logic paper, "Fuzzy Sets," argues that "we do manipulate information . . . but the objects of our reason are generally not [binary] numbers but fuzzy patterns without sharply defined boundaries" (1965).

By using this perspective, I will question polarized, bounded, all-or-nothing linguistic categorizations of sexual behaviors such as safety/danger, unsafe/safe(r), relapser/nonrelapser, lapser/nonlapser, nature/nurture, rational/irrational, and I will *somewhat* critique health education interventions premised upon such binary categories and *somewhat* applaud those that are not.

To put it briefly, pleasurable and sexual realities for the individual, I suggest, are fluid in both time and space, not rigid or easily classified into "sharply defined boundaries." Dichotomous categorizations distort sexual realities as well as the meaning and sensuousness of real-life sexual experiences. In other words, in regard to sexual (and perhaps many other) behaviors, human beings do not obey binary rules and do not fit into neatly labeled boxes as their situations and sexual behaviors change through time, reeling into one another, as one context blends into another.

I realize this will be unsettling for some. My arguments in the final two chapters will undoubtedly invite disdain from those who venerate all-or-nothing categories into which sexual behaviors must fit.

Part of this response occurs by virtue of the nature of disorder itself, that gray amorphous mass between and/or beyond discretely ordered categories such as unsafe/safe(r) or rational/irrational. Disorder is unlimited and to date remains an area of human experience for which no pattern yet exists.

And, of course, humans crave pattern, design, or order over chaos and disorder. Disorder represents unknown danger, disorder provokes discomfort. More than a decade ago, anthropologist Mary Douglas advanced the notion that disorder is "dangerous" because it breaks down existing patterns or categories, but, at the same time, it is powerful because it has "potentiality" (1966). The gray, shifting zones of an individual's life experience, including those murky areas of sexual pleasure and desire, are where power—the power to dispel extreme categories—and potential—the potential to understand—lie waiting.

My research for this book took place in West Hollywood, California in 1993–94. West Hollywood, covering approximately two square miles, is quaintly nestled between the wealthy city of Beverly Hills to the west and the once glamorous Hollywood district of Los Angeles to the east. It is the major of two gay and lesbian meccas in the Los Angeles area where multiple business establishments cater to a gay and lesbian clientele and where a gay culture continues to flourish despite the modern HIV plague (Gorman 1992). In West Hollywood, professional men and women, blue-collar workers, gay and lesbian mothers and fathers all go about their everyday lives as do citizens in any American community. They shop at the local grocery store, visit the hardware store to purchase tools and home repair goods, eat out at their favorite restaurants.

However, bonded by adversity, this is also a community rich with colorful ritualistic cultural celebrations. Every June, for example, a four- to six-hour parade exuberantly marches down Santa Monica Boulevard, the main West Hollywood strip. The parade is part of a nationwide celebration of Gay Pride Month. Besides thousands of individuals, dozens of businesses, politicians, community and activist groups such as the Gay Democrats, Gay Republicans, Parents and Friends of Lesbians and Gays (P-FLAG), Gay Fathers, ACT-UP, and Gay and Lesbian Teachers, to name only a few, take part, winding along the strip in a carnival-like atmosphere. Businesses and politicians frequently use this opportunity to show their support for the gay community and to market their particular services or to gain gay and lesbian votes. The strip's bars and businesses become packed with gay folk as Santa Monica Boulevard becomes one gigantic party.

Every year the parade thematically emphasizes and extols the role of eroticism in gay culture. Floats pass by carrying muscular men dancing in G-strings while the spectators themselves, wearing the skimpiest of clothing or flamboyantly adorned (or both), tan their athletic bodies in the hot June sun. Occasionally, some of the women will remove their tops and join their male counterparts to freely cavort bare-breasted beneath the sun's rays. A few parade marchers dance and swirl, tossing condoms—the emblem of safe(r) sex—into the crowd like ticker tape streamers.

In addition to the parade, a festival is held for the entire weekend, with plenty of food, drink (alcoholic and non), crafts, and other wares offered for sale. At each end of a city park (which serves as festival grounds), makeshift, tented dance floors are set up so that revelers can lightly trip the two-step to a country and western twang or dance themselves into a trance to the pounding beat of disco and contemporary industrial rock. In the disco tent especially, the majority of dancers are shirtless and sweaty as the atmosphere takes on a palpable, surging carnality. Bending and twisting to the music's pulsing rhythm, men kiss and rub their bodies together; one man's rotating pelvis moves in sensual synchronicity with another's undulating buttocks as they lick and embrace in an erotic ritual of sensuality, all the while lost in the constant "boom boom boom" of the music's relentless bass.

In recent years, the festival has become an arena for local AIDS organizations to offer safer sex demonstrations and to recruit people into safer sex workshops. As an ominous sign of the times, medical groups, home health care companies, and even funeral homes have begun to open booths at similar events around the country.

West Hollywood is also the scene for another major ritualistic celebration of gay culture—Halloween. On Halloween night, October 31, Santa Monica Boulevard is closed to traffic and the busy thoroughfare once again becomes a showcase for parades of outrageously costumed celebrants. Haughty drag queens in imperious excess and beautiful young men in clinging loincloths or revealing Roman garb dance and carouse through the awestruck crowd. People flow in and out of the bars and shops, and stages for music and comedy performances are set up on each end of the strip. Groups of costumed merrymakers perform skits in the middle of the crowded boulevard, drawing laughter as flocks of pseudo-nuns whisk by on skates through the merry maze. And, if revelers are lucky, they will catch a glimpse of the West Hollywood Cheerleaders.

The West Hollywood Cheerleaders are a group of about a half dozen men who dress in red and white female cheerleading outfits, complete with pleated skirts and pullover sweaters embossed with the giant red letters W and H across their gargantuan fake breasts. Constantly waving red-and-white pom-poms and blowing kisses to doting admirers, the "girls" sport wigs that are sometimes teased at least a foot high. The Cheerleaders are mascots of the town and often appear at fund-raisers to help in the fight against AIDS and to benefit other gay and lesbian causes.

Although for more than a decade HIV has hit the gay population relentlessly, the community as a whole appears to have maintained its sense of humor and ability to laugh at itself and others. Even in a city oppressed by grief and tragedy in the midst of one of history's most hideous epidemics, life goes on and individuals prosper despite the shattering loss of citizens, friends, and lovers to AIDS.

My methodological approach to this project is both qualitative and ethnographic. While living in West Hollywood, I gathered data through my participation in two health education and prevention programs targeting gay men who had "difficulty" maintaining safer sex practices. I also ran two focus groups on the topic and conducted separate in-depth unstructured interviews of thirty gay men, mostly Caucasian or Hispanic, who lived in or frequented West Hollywood. Sometimes the interview took place over two visits, sometimes only one. However, to gain a deeper understanding of the HIV-negative gay man's experience, I interviewed one individual informant during multiple sessions over a five-week period.

I limited the study to HIV-negative gay men, aged thirty to forty-four. In a large survey of gay and bisexual men living in the Los Angeles metropolitan area, this age group reportedly was more likely to have had a recent experience of anal sex without a condom (Kanouse et al. 1991). Moreover, I thought men in this age group would possess a longer, richer experience living as gay-identified men in the days before and after HIV/AIDS announced its presence. It was more than conceivable that they would have suffered a greater sense of loss than their younger counterparts. Finally, this age group makes up a cultural cohort, a group of men who came out after the Stonewall riots and grew out of the gay sexual revolution and political activism of the 1970s (Herdt and Boxer 1991).

To be completely accurate (but to spare those readers who cringe at the sight of a chart), I have provided additional details about the entire research project—including sample demographics, aggregate descriptive data, and comments on the limitations of the study itself—in appendixes A and B at the end of the book. In appendix A, I also include a brief discussion of qualitative research methods. However, given that focus groups are currently in vogue both among researchers and program planners—and for readers who for one reason or another choose to skip the appendixes—I will take a moment here to outline the problems associated with the use of this data collection method for understanding private sexual behaviors.

Focus groups are usually of little value in exploring taboo topics (Scrimshaw and Hurtado 1987). The focus group participants in my study were unwilling to talk about their own experiences with unprotected anal sex and spent much of the hour and a half discussion time in hypothesizing about why "other" gay men might indulge in such behaviors. At the end of the session, however, participants filled out a short and private questionnaire. Not too surprisingly, the questionnaire data show a different reality than do the data from the focus groups. (An AIDS activist friend of mine calls this kind of research "Tah Dah" research, meaning that the answer is obvious before the research begins.)

In the first of the two focus groups, over half the participants reported on the postgroup questionnaire that they had had anal sex without a condom in the last year. In this same group, only one of the seven participants admitted to this practice during the discussion period. When this lone man shared his experience with the other group participants, his voice wavered and his face flushed. One of the other participants shook his head, pursed his lips, and glared at the confessor with contempt. The man who was candid about this sexual act now became socially polluted in the eyes of the other participants. On the other hand, oral sex without a condom, a community norm, was discussed openly and freely with much enthusiasm by all participants as they shared their literal distaste for performing fellatio on a latex-shrouded penis.

The most obvious explanation for the contrast in response to these differing behaviors is that using a condom for anal sex represents the ideal norm among gay men (Kelly et al. 1991; Kelly, Lawrence, and Brasfield 1991). Social norms can be maintained through shame (as well as by positive reinforcement) if the behavior is a public one—but sex is usually a private behavior. Shame can nonetheless have an subversive impact on private sexual behaviors: an individual may continue to perform the behavior in private but just not admit it in public. For a gay man to admit publicly that he did not use a condom during an anal sex experience would bring him shame, stigma, sometimes even a harsh reprimand from other gay men, whether HIV-infected or not, and certainly disapprobation from health educators (Odets 1995). Consequently, to avoid shame, gay men may not discuss their private sexual behaviors in a focus group that is likely to include judgmental others.

Clearly, focus groups have severe limitations when used in sexual behavior research. This type of research requires a more private, anonymous and/or confidential approach whether the research is qualitative or quantitative. In the present study, along with the focus groups I used one-on-one, face-to-face, qualitative interviews. The interviews were private and confidential, and in contrast with the focus groups, the men shared not only their oral sex encounters but also many details about their anal sex experiences without condoms.

There is, of course, more to the men interviewed than just their sexual experiences. Although I explored the complexity of their lives in my interviews, the focus here will be on sexual experiences and sexual lives. However, this should not lead the reader to stereotype gay men as strictly sexual beings. Just as with most people, regardless of sexuality, sex is just one facet of these men's lives, albeit an important one (Browning 1994). Moreover, instead of highlighting one history or only presenting an analysis in the aggregate, I chose to present six separate case studies from the interviews. Five cases are of single men, and one case is made up of a pair of "monogamous" lovers. I sought to select men who best expressed the themes representative of the diversity of the men sampled (see appendix B). All but two of the men in the chosen interviews had had at least one experience the previous year in which he and/or his partner did not wear a condom for anal sex.

Given the sensitive and confidential nature of the topic, I do not, of course, give their real names. (In any case, since the men were allowed to use a pseudonym, I may not even have this knowledge.) Additionally, I have sometimes, with much reluctance, left out information or changed the names of places not pertinent to the topic at hand if I felt it was possible that such information might reveal an individual's identity. In doing so, I balance accuracy with ethical concerns.

Before presenting these accounts, however, I give in chapter 1 a brief history of HIV prevention, describe current issues surrounding gay men and the maintenance of unsafe(r) sex, and provide an interpretive framework using fuzzy logic. Following this, I move on to chapter 2, a love story, the story of Johnny and Ralph. Although they are enamored, they have different erotic needs. Ralph wants to maintain a monogamous relationship, but Johnny has other fantasies to which he occasionally succumbs. Their story provides some understanding of sexual (mis)communication between two men in a "monogamous" relationship.

Chapter 3 tells the story of Bob, a business consultant who found out about my project through an announcement placed in a newsletter at an AIDS organization where he volunteers as a caregiver. Bob says that he always uses a condom for anal sex but draws the line when it comes to oral sex, which he practices without a condom. For Bob oral sex is a risk-reduction strategy, not a risky behavior.

In Chapter 4, I introduce Phil. He is afraid of HIV infection, and he is afraid of himself. Fear and guilt drive Phil to go for long periods of practicing masturbation to the backdrop of pornographic films. These periods are punctuated with episodes of anal sex, sometimes without a condom. Phil's pornography seems to replace his desire for sexual encounters, and he spends many an evening masturbating to the groans emanating from his television's stereo sound. But sometimes "the porno just doesn't cut it" and Phil wants more. So he ventures out into the West Hollywood night to search for a sexual partner. On one such occasion, he becomes a performer in a real-life version of one of his favorite erotic fantasies.

Chapter 5 recounts the story of Alexander. Alexander does not know how he could be capable of having anal sex without a condom—which he did in the month before the interview—especially since he is an HIV social service professional. Unlike the other cases presented here, I knew Alexander before his interview, at least in passing. He called me after seeing the green flyers distributed to recruit study participants (see appendix B). He believed he could contribute "something of value" to the study, but I was somewhat hesitant and concerned that our limited acquaintance might inhibit his sharing of any experiences about which he may have felt shame. As it turned out, this was not a problem.

In contrast, Roger, in chapter 6, hesitated to share his sexual experiences with me despite the fact that I was a stranger to him. At the age of thirty, he is the youngest man in the study and came out as a gay man at a time when HIV was already ravaging the gay community. He once felt cheated for not having experienced anal sex without a condom, and he envied his older counterparts who were sexually active before AIDS. He was curious about what unprotected anal sex must be like. Now that he has had such an experience, however, his curiosity has gone through a psychological metamorphosis, transforming into guilt.

The last case study is Jerry, a nurse. Jerry describes himself as a "top leather man," meaning that he likes wearing black leather attire when he goes out to the bars or likes to wear/use leather accoutrement when having "masculine sex." He insists on being the "top" or penetrator during anal sex because he likes to be the one in control of his sexual encounters, but one night in October 1993, in his own words, he "lost control."

These are the HIV-negative men whose stories make up this book. All have had a lengthy and intense experience with AIDS. Several of their friends and acquaintances have fallen to the disease, and some continue to volunteer and to work with people with AIDS. Despite these semblances, they are diverse in their childhood experiences, various relationships, sexual histories and fantasies, coping strategies, views on what it means to be gay, and what sexual practices really turn them on. Yet most had had anal sex without a condom at least once in the not-too-distant past.

These men are the ones that educators and researchers sometimes say "should know better." Indeed, they should and they do. But knowledge and experience alone cannot prevent the occurrence of unsafer sex (Joseph et al. 1987a, 1987b; McCusker et al. 1989; Siegel et al. 1988). It takes more, much more, as the upcoming stories so tellingly demonstrate.

In the final two chapters I apply fuzzy logic to an evolutionary analysis of unsafer sex and put human sexual pleasure within the theoretical context of interactions between biology, the environment, psychology, social relations, and culture. In this overarching context, I will, in the end, make suggestions for HIV prevention education, using an existing Los Angeles program as an exemplar.

I wrote this book in the hope that it would appeal to a variety of readers, yet I recognize that not everyone shares the same interests. Although many readers will want to explore the work in its entirety, some will undoubtedly choose to skip the opening chapter as well as the more theoretical final chapters altogether (or read them later), preferring instead to move directly to the sexual life histories. I find this approach completely understandable.

And although some (or perhaps many) will disagree partially or wholeheartedly with my theoretical framework and perspectives, I write this book in unison with my critics. For despite our differing points of view, we are all committed to the ongoing and relentless struggle against the AIDS epidemic. I trust this book will make a contribution toward this effort.

Risky Sex

1

History, Risky Sex, and Relapse

To give up on understanding sex is to surrender to ignorance, to despair of our own potential for thought and knowledge.

—Dean Hamer and Peter Copeland, *The Science of Desire* (1994)

Having failed to suppress forbidden desire, modern society has elected to isolate and assign it to a distant category of "other" people.

—G. Browning, *The Culture of Desire* (1994)

Last dance, last chance for love.

—"Last Dance," as sung by Donna Summer

Contentious Virus

The 1969 Stonewall riots in New York's Greenwich Village marked a move from private sexual identity to public sexual identity, a move from homosexual to gay (Herdt and Boxer 1991), and in the 1970s gay men who lived in or who frequented large urban areas in the United States were indeed, in the literal sense, "gay." Many migrated to urban settings where they found more freedom, acceptance, sex, and community. They "came out of the closet," performing a cultural rite of passage by announcing their gay identity to relatives, friends, and to the public. They were proud to be gay, and gay and lesbian cultural institutions and celebrations flourished (Herdt 1992; Herdt and Boxer 1991; Herrel 1992; Murray 1992; Sedgewick 1990).

No one suspected that an infectious agent, Human Immunodeficiency Virus (HIV), was lurking among the beds, bars, bathrooms, bookstores, and bathhouses of major urban centers. Sex was free, liberated, pleasurable, and erotic, and it was a time for male sexual experimentation. It was a time for venereal diseases too, but no one

seemed to mind since penicillin, one of the wonders of modern medicine, tended to take care of that loathsome little inconvenience
(Shilts 1987).

In the early 1980s, however, whispers swirled through smoke-
filled gay bars, breaking the syncopated sip-sip-sip emanating from
cocktail glasses and bottles of politically correct beers. (Certain beer
brands were boycotted because their owners were known or thought
to be antigay.) Patrons exchanged tempered concerns about a new illness, an illness that at that time carried the label of "gay cancer." Was
it real? Was it some cancer caused perhaps by the teensy brown bottles of amyl nitrate ("poppers"), held between thumb and forefinger
to the nose, spreading its locker room scent above the nightly flash-
ing disco light shows and used to heighten the same-sex carnal
encounters so relished in New York, Los Angeles, and San Francisco?
The whispers whirled, rising with fear as more and more young men
succumbed to the unforeseen modern-day plague. Some gay men
thought the so-called cancer to be nothing more than a plot concocted by a homophobic society to quash their newly found sexual
liberation while other men began to sweat, especially at night, as
their fevers soared and the once foreign but now all-too-familiar
raised purple lesions of Kaposi's sarcoma ravaged their skin (Kramer
1989; Shilts 1987).

Eventually, researchers changed the disease's label from the vague
"gay cancer" to Gay Related Immune Deficiency (GRID), then later
on, with the urging of hemophiliacs, global scientists, and others, the
disease earned yet another name, now engraved in history, of Acquired Immune Deficiency Syndrome (AIDS).

In 1983 both Luc Montagnier of France and Robert Gallo of the
United States claimed to have isolated the virus causing this new
affliction (Barre-Sinoussi et al. 1983; Gallo et al. 1984). Amid a storm
of scientific controversy, as both researchers publicly brawled over
who had actually discovered this strange microbe, Margaret Heckler,
then U.S. Secretary of Health and Human Services, held a press conference on April 23, 1984, to announce that Robert Gallo had detected
the virus that causes AIDS. Those aware of the politics of HIV were
not surprised that Heckler did not mention Luc Montagnier's name.
In spite of this international scientific furor, gay men gave a collective
sigh of relief in the false belief that the end to their plague was near.

Soon, some thought, HIV would mean little more than a visit to the neighborhood clinic for a vaccine shot (Panem 1988; Shilts 1987).

While gay men rushed to embrace a newfound optimism, the bitter dispute between Gallo and Montagnier took on political dimensions as each side, supported by his own respective national research enterprises, persisted; lawyers were kept busy filing lawsuits and countersuits over the right to patent an antibodies test for HIV. In time an international settlement was reached and an HIV test eventually became available, but this only increased the calls warning against potential government lists of the infected and of those suspected of being infected (Panem 1988; Shilts 1987).

The Gay Muses and the Public's Health

Early in the epidemic, even before the availability of HIV testing, the gay community had mobilized. Gay men, lesbians, and their friends and supporters formed groups such as Los Angeles Shanti and AIDS Project Los Angeles (APLA) in order to provide sanity, hope, and conviction in the midst of alarm. One of the original activists involved in the founding of APLA, Tom Mosley, recounts those early days.

> I was at the Probe [a Los Angeles gay bar] when I first heard stories about a gay cancer. Homosexuals all over New York City were falling to this surrealistic ailment. It had also shown up in San Francisco. And, quite recently, one of our own Probe members had become a victim of this peculiar syndrome. Suddenly, the back bar became a clearing house for medical information. And it was in this unlikely venue that I recollect seeing the first organized effort to lay the cornerstone of the project [APLA].
>
> (quoted in Furin 1995:282)

The project itself began in 1983 as an information hotline operating out of a tiny apartment on Cole Avenue in the center of Hollywood. Today APLA is one of the largest AIDS service organizations in the United States, with an annual budget of around $20 million. APLA provides case management, treatment advocacy, dental care, food, psychosocial support services, home health care, and last but not least, prevention education. In the beginning, however, the operation had consisted of a mere handful of dedicated individuals seeking to bring sanity and compassion into the dark maze of uncertainty and hysteria (Furin 1995).

Once epidemiologists and other researchers had determined that AIDS was a sexually transmitted disease, a few prevention education programs received a funding boost. Gay pundits like activist Cleve Jones in San Francisco and playwright Larry Kramer in New York had already indicted "homosexual hypersexuality" and "exotic" sexual practices such as anal sex, fisting (slowly inserting a fist into another person's anus), and rimming (licking another person's anus) as the "cause" of AIDS. Larry Kramer preached like a messianic Cassandra, shouting his warning message, a message that at that time was largely ignored.

Soon Don Francis and others from the Centers for Disease Control (CDC) joined the gay muses as they warned their gay brethren to "sexually slow down," but government involvement, welcomed by some, fueled the anger of the gay conspiracy theorists and sexual liberation activists who denounced the CDC's efforts as homophobic. They insisted that the accompanying public health calls to close gay bathhouses were only the beginning of attempts to turn back the sexual and political clock to the 1950s and to force gays back into the closet (Kramer 1989; Shilts 1987).

The Religious Right

As the gay community continued to mobilize, and as the international battle over who had discovered the virus causing AIDS persisted, and while the government diddled, the religious right in America was unleashing its fearful and hateful dogma. According to this view, AIDS is the result of God's wrath, a curse on the "sinful and unnatural" behaviors of gay men. To those in the religious right, this is God's retribution; by bringing down "homosexual sinners," God is doing something they feel is necessary and just. As one member of the Pro-Family Christian Coalition in Reno, Nevada, put it, "I think we should do what the Bible says, and cut their [gay men's] throats" (Altman 1986:68). Somewhat contradictorily, people dying of cancer and other potentially fatal diseases are not necessarily on God's hit list; this is, apparently, just their bad luck.

The media rallied in the right wing's shadow, feeding a frenzy of public fear (Albert 1986). America plummeted into a state of moral panic, and to some people all gay men became dangerous and contagious suspects (Watney 1988). In 1984, Republican Congressman William Dannemeyer launched a California ballot initiative to quarantine anyone "suspected" of HIV infection (*read* gay men). Some gay men in Los Angeles, as I recall, seriously considered leaving the country, but the referendum failed to pass after two attempts thanks to the combined political muscle of the gay community, public health experts, and medical professionals (Bayer 1989; Shilts 1987).

But despite this onslaught of ignorance from the religious right and their discriminatory politico-religious abominations, gay men and others who preferred facts over irrational hatred now knew what caused AIDS. They knew how it was transmitted. They could take a test to identify possible infection. Along with this information, however, came one of the most momentous challenges in the legacy of gay-identified men: they had to learn to adapt to their deadly and infectious viral neighbor. This situation required behavioral change on a massive scale.

Health Education and Relapse

In the early to mid-1980s, generally conservative social mores, petty politics, and calcified religious beliefs continued to stifle efforts to obtain outside assistance for programs to enact behavioral change. Right-wing politicians, arguing that such prevention programs would foster promiscuity and promote a "homosexual lifestyle," effectively blocked government-funded HIV prevention programs or diluted them with severe content restrictions (Bayer 1989). As a result, most gay men, with the help of some adventurous and progressive community organizations, were left to cope on their own and to find ways to change their behaviors. For some, this meant seeking refuge in a monogamous relationship. For others, it meant reducing their number of sexual partners. For a small group, it meant abstinence, at least temporarily, while other gay men began to use condoms for the first time (Martin 1986).

Once public health HIV prevention campaigns did kick off in the mid to late 1980s, they were primarily based upon social marketing theory and upon traditional public health models such as the Health Belief Model, the theory of reasoned action, and other similar knowledge-based approaches (Levinton 1989; Martin 1986; Valdiserri et al. 1989; Williams 1986). Earlier programs leaned toward promoting abstinence and reducing the number of sexual partners but also touted the use of condoms. How much or how little these programs actually accomplished in prompting behavioral change is a matter of debate (Gold 1993). At the very least, however, these interventions did teach some gay men important basic facts concerning AIDS, and for the first time they learned how to put on a condom *properly*—no small matter.

Nonetheless, whatever the "real" cause of the behavior change— whether through public health education, self-motivation, personal experience, word-of-mouth, or all of the above—American gay men, on the whole, did change their behavior and condom use became for the most part widespread (Becker and Joseph 1988; Joseph et al. 1987a, 1987b; Martin 1986; McCusker et al. 1989; McKusick et al. 1985; McKusick et al. 1990; Stall, Coates, and Hoff 1988; and Valdiserri et al. 1989).

Starting in the 1990s, however, this pattern of safer sexual behavior appeared to be undergoing a process of change. Although the rate of HIV seroconversion has decreased among gay men as a whole, in one study of 479 men in four cities, 47 percent of the gay respondents reported unprotected anal intercourse in the previous six months (Kelly et al. 1991). Similar findings abound in the AIDS-prevention literature, with multiple studies sounding the alarm that gay men are returning to unsafer sex (see Adib et al. 1991; Ekstrand and Coates 1990; McCusker et al. 1992; Stall et al. 1990). Moreover, this phenomenon is not limited to gay men living in the United States but is shared with gay men in Europe, Australia, and New Zealand (de Wit, Van Den Hock et al. 1993; de Wit, Van Griensven et al. 1993; Gold 1995; Kippax et al. 1993).

Within the geographic area where the men interviewed for this book reside, a Los Angeles county survey of gay and bisexual men sponsored by the Rand Corporation found that only 31 percent of 285 gay men who defined themselves as "sexually active" said that they use condoms "all the time" (Kanouse et al. 1991:26). This state of affairs has left many health educators, researchers, therapists, health care providers, and gay men frustrated and demoralized. Some are afraid that most Americans will say, "Gay men should know better. If they get infected, it's their own damn fault." One health educator in Los Angeles expressed his uneasiness to me this way: "I guess there's just this fringe we'll never reach. I don't know what their problem is and we've done all we can. It makes us [gay men] look bad. I just don't know why they [other gay men] put themselves at risk? . . . Maybe low self-esteem, feeling guilty about not being infected [with HIV], who knows for sure?"

Beneath this educator's frustration lies an erroneous assumption: obviously, based upon the studies I just mentioned, we are not talking about a fringe population. The numbers are too large and the individuals are not geographically isolated. Additionally, he identifies a couple of the various reasons given by researchers and professionals for the increase in unsafer sex practices among gay men. I'll discuss these in detail shortly, but first, in order to avoid ambiguity and misunderstanding, some basic terms used in health education and research (and the heated controversy surrounding their application) warrant clarification.

Few concepts, with the exception of the term *risk groups* (groups with high incidence and prevalence of HIV infection), have stirred more interdisciplinary controversy in this area of research than the term *relapse*. Relapse, technically defined, simply means giving up a newly acquired healthy behavior and returning to an old unhealthy behavior. The fields of public health and social psychology have used the relapse construct for quite some time to categorize those people who have difficulty staying on a diet, giving up smoking and alcohol, and the like (Levinton 1989; Schunk and Carbonari 1984). Once public health workers and social psychologists applied the relapse label to giving up safer sex, scholars quickly responded, some with an acidic tongue and others with less stringent reconceptualizations.

Probably the most cynical idea floating about in regard to the relapse concept is based upon "self-interest theory." Relapse, so states the theory, was introduced into safer sex by educators and researchers who wanted to save their jobs. After all, the argument goes, if gay men stopped having unsafer sex, what would those self-interested educators and researchers do for a living? Given the political reality that prevention funding has not created a wealth of dollars and is subject to change at political whim, the theory is not well-founded (see Hart et al. 1992).

In addition, based upon my experience working in health education as an educator, researcher, and program evaluator, I find the suggestion of self-interest motivation—bordering on a vulgar conspiracy—implausible for numerous other reasons. It ignores the fact that many educators are volunteers, and it brushes aside the day-to-day reality that some health educators and researchers employed in HIV pay a price, a price of stigma. HIV educators may not tell their relatives, for example, what kind of work they do, and if they do tell, their friends and relatives would, as one educator told me, "rather not discuss IT [meaning AIDS]. My mother lies and tells people I work with the handicapped. Something more noble. Something with a little less stigma attached." Moreover, advocates of the self-interest theory assume that AIDS educators and researchers could not find jobs elsewhere (perhaps with better pay, fewer hours, and unquestionably with less outside criticism and scrutiny), and they disregard the choices made by some educators and researchers to abandon more lucrative careers in order to work for "the cause."

There are, of course, other and fairer critiques of relapse. Some of these have come from researchers in England, Europe, and Australia. Hart et al. (1992) of the United Kingdom, for example, find the "static" concept of relapse to be overly medical and unnecessary at this stage of the epidemic. They worry about the consequences, both political and personal, of applying the relapse construct to gay men, arguing that

> what we see here, therefore, is an account of male sexuality—incorporating hetero- and homo-sexual behaviour—which is dependent on penetration, urges or needs that are inherently difficult to control, and the inevitability of return [relapse] to given forms of sexual expression in the absence of thorough, consistent and long-term policing. This conceptual admixture of disease presence, remission, back sliding, addiction and the inevitability of unrestricted penetration in male sexuality is a combination which, when applied to populations of gay men, further reinforces their otherness as outsiders marked by perversion [disease] and sexual appetites of heroic proportions. Such a con-

struction of gay men cannot be useful in any attempts to help them find ways to protect themselves from a life-threatening and sexually transmitted infection.   (1992:227)

Detractors of this argument submit that it is too "preliminary" to make such claims (Donovan et al. 1995). They find suspected rein-forcement of negative attitudes regarding gay men and gay sex by the use of the term *relapse* to be theoretically interesting but contend that it has not been demonstrated to be the case factually. At this stage, it is conjecture.

Instead of hypothesizing possible consequences of the term's application, researchers from the Netherlands and Australia have defined what does and does not constitute relapse, and in doing so have contributed a much needed (though still insufficient) refine-ment of the relapse construct. These researchers, distinguishing re-lapsers from lapsers, define relapse in the traditional sense—as a *con-sistent* return to risky sex. Lapsers, on the other hand, are individuals who *occasionally* engage in unsafer sex. Using this distinction, they have found that relapsers are more likely to be gay men in a relation-ship with a man of the same serostatus whereas lapsers are less likely to be in a relationship (de Wit, Van Den Hock et al. 1993; de Wit, Van Griensven et al. 1993; Kippax et al. 1993).

In this book I am sympathetic to the perception that the relapse label has been misused, but the term *lapser* also bears limitations for determining risk and requires a "fuzzier" differentiation. Although lapser is an improvement, both *lapser* and *relapser* are based on a worldview that may not fit the reality of individual sexual lives which are fluid in both time and space.

During a sexual life history, for instance, an individual usually moves from one category to another, with transitions of safer sex in between. A relapser may fade into becoming a lapser who fades into practicing consistent safer sex, then move again to lapser (or re-lapser), back to relapser (or lapser), and so on throughout his life-time. He may move in and out of relationships, changing his condom use practices depending upon the HIV status of his partner(s) at the time and the length of the relationship. The overall time period of any given survey measurement (six months, one year, four years, and so on) determines the label that researchers place on him.

To illustrate the point, suppose that one measures a man's condom use while he is in a relationship: when having sex within the relationship he uses a condom, but says he only sometimes uses a condom when he has sex outside the relationship. Is he a relapser or nonrelapser? What if he does not use a condom in the relationship but always or sometimes uses one while having sex with men outside the relationship? Is he a lapser or a relapser? After he leaves a relationship in which he only practiced unprotected sex, at what point does he become a nonrelapser? Three months later? Six months later? One year later? If, after the relationship ended, he has thirty different sexual encounters in a one-year period and only one, the fifteenth encounter, was unprotected, is he a lapser? Or is he a nonrelapser since the last fifteen encounters were all protected? If six months ago he had unsafer sex once and then during the next six months only has safer sex, at what point did he become a nonrelapser? Or is he still a lapser? Is the glass half empty or is the glass half full? Or, as Kosko has asked (as pointed out in my introduction), where does an apple in the process of being eaten "cross the line from apple to nonapple?" (1993:4).

Relapser and lapser labels present the same problem as does Kosko's apple/nonapple dilemma. These labels may be useful linguistic devices, but they tell us little about individual sexual patterns, sexual context, and decision-making processes through time. For the present volume, owing to the state of the research record, I will use these labels while discussing other researchers' works. But I will abandon them later on in my final analysis.

There remains yet one important area of confusion about the relapse construct that I will now attempt to make clear, and that is the specific sexual behaviors researchers and educators are talking about when using the relapse label. Most studies define relapse and lapse in relation to the nonuse of a condom for anogenital sex, while a few have lumped together unprotected oral and anal sex without a condom (see Donovan et al. 1995; Hospers and Kok 1995). To combine oral sex and anal sex into a single category is decidedly unscientific and definitely provides more of an example of fuzzy thinking than it does of fuzzy logic. Oral sex without a condom is much less risky than anal sex without a condom (Ostrow et al. 1995), and a man's reason for engaging in "unprotected" oral sex may be quite different from those for engaging in unprotected anal sex. Moreover, it could just as well be argued that replacing unprotected anal sex with unprotected oral sex is a real risk-reduction strategy. Although I will elaborate further on this matter in the last two chapters, from this point on, when I refer to the terms *relapse* or *lapser*, I am restricting their meanings unequivocally to the practice of unprotected anal sex.

Some researchers have ventured to find or build a consensus about why some men return to the practice of anogenital sex sans condom, but more often than not, they end up uncovering multiple and often contradictory answers to an intensely complex question. The earliest surveys of gay men returning to risky sex were longitudinal studies in San Francisco, during which, before collecting their data, researchers had made no distinction between lapsers and relapsers. For example, Stall and his colleagues (1990) kept track of 397 San Francisco gay men for two years. For these men, several factors were found to be associated with a return to unsafer sex, including a "preference" for sex without a condom; however, the researchers also noted that results varied based upon the study participant's relationship with his partner. Those men who enjoyed a relationship with a lover were likely not to use a condom for anal sex because they were in love and knew their partner's HIV status. Those men not in a relationship reported sexual arousal as a key reason for unprotected sex.

Another longitudinal study of 686 gay men in the same city suggested that a "return" to risky sex was associated with a younger age, more sexual partners, having had no experience of losing friends or lovers to AIDS, and with not engaging in other questionable health behaviors (Ekstrand and Coates 1990). And in a 1991 six-month retrospective study of 470 men in four U.S. cities (Memphis, Tampa, Mobile, and Binghamton), "relapsers" expressed having affectionate feelings for a partner, wanting to please a partner, having a negative attitude toward condoms, and "being caught in the moment" as reasons for resorting to unsafer sex (Kelly et al. 1991).

In 1993 a few European and Australian research articles on relapse were published in AIDS-related journals. After making a distinction between lapsers (occasional unsafer sex) and relapsers (consistent unsafe sex), they found that "true" relapsers who "never" used a condom were more likely to be in a relationship with someone of the same serostatus—in other words, an HIV-negative man with an HIV-negative man or an HIV-positive man with an HIV-positive man. Lapsers, on the other hand, tended to have less positive attitudes about condoms, less intention to avoid unprotected anal sex, and lower personal efficacy with respect to using condoms with "casual" partners. Lapsers, however, aware of the risk involved with their behavior (Bosga et al. 1995; de Wit, Van Griensven et al. 1993; de Wit, Van Den Hock et al. 1993; Kippax et al. 1993).

As if this confusion were not enough, Walt Odets (1995), a psychotherapist, claims that HIV-negative gay men may participate in unsafe sex out of "survivor guilt." Gay men, the theory goes, have a conscious or unconscious desire to become infected because of their guilt for being healthy. Odets writes:

> Because AIDS is such an available and psychologically meaningful way for a gay man to not survive, it is surprising how difficult it has been for us to acknowledge that some men engage in unprotected sex for precisely that purpose. There are many psychologically intelligible reasons men might not wish to survive the AIDS epidemic. They include depression, anxiety, and guilt, including guilt about surviving; lives emptied by loss, isolation, and loneliness; the loss of social affiliation and psychological identity; and anticipation of a future that holds more of the same.
>
> (1995:206)

There is no doubt that HIV-negative gay men have suffered exceedingly and continue to suffer sometimes overwhelming feelings of sorrow and grief at the loss of friends and lovers from AIDS, but I remain skeptical (though not close-minded) about this rather bleak and gloomy theory.

In a somewhat related idea, some educators believe that gay men engage in unsafer sex due to their low self-esteem or from a low value of self fostered by the stigma attached to growing up with gay feelings and the devaluation of homosexuality in many cultures. This attribute can only be "corrected" or converted into its opposite—high self-esteem—by way of therapy or by various "feel good" interventions (Dawes 1994; Torey 1972). As one educator in Los Angeles told me, "If we can just get them to feel good instead of bad about themselves, they'll be all right. They've been told that they are inherently bad, so of course they do bad things" (also see Odets 1995).

The use of the self-esteem construct is problematical. It is unclear in research results, for example, if "low self-esteem" causes a behavior or is caused by the behavior itself. Thus one may have a temporary feeling of low self-esteem because one has performed an act which broke a social norm (e.g., anal sex without a condom) instead of incurring the supposed and more inherent low self-esteem deemed to be causing the act.

Moreover, the whole notion of self-esteem is built upon a cultural assumption of a cohesive self and a self valuation which may not be valid. According to Katherine Ewing, "At any particular moment a person usually experiences his or her articulated self as symbolic, but this self may be quickly displaced by another, quite different 'self', which is based on a different definition of the situation" (1990:251). In other words, self-esteem is a fuzzy construct, and one's degree of self-esteem may vary across time and place. Just because one has a lower value of self due to one's oppression or childhood experiences does not mean this lower value is present in all situations—including sexual ones—at all times.

Nevertheless, I will share gay men's tales of anguish, guilt, and their self valuation in the coming interviews as coping with death, grief, and oppression do play a prominent role in gay men's lives and in their responses to an unsafer sexual encounter. But I will also insist that any theory of unsafer sex, at least when sex is consensual and not coerced, must figure pleasure into the causal equation.

Given the plethora of theories, it appears that there is much disagreement about why gay men continue to practice or sometimes return to unsafer sex, but there is one exceptional area of majority agreement among both educators and researchers. Most agree that men in lover relationships who have the same HIV status prefer not to use a condom when having sex as a couple because unprotected anal penetration is pleasurable and is a way of expressing intimacy. In support of this, a qualitative study in Norway provides some descriptive data on the importance of anal sex for gay men. In that study, Prieur (1990) suggests that accepting semen without a condom is a way of showing love and affection, and failure to ejaculate inside a partner is a sign of a holding back of self. In other words, for men in relationships, semen is not seen as dangerous but rather as something special, a gift of love and intimacy.

The consensus is only limited, however, to an explanation as to why gay men have unprotected sex, not to the safety of their behavior. Some researchers reason that the discontinuance of condom use by men in monogamous relationships where both partners have the same serostatus is safe. They brand the lovers' behaviors as "negotiated safety" (Kippax et al. 1993). Detractors point out that monogamy is an ideal from which one of the partners may stray without telling the other. This camp also argues that a man may not reveal his real HIV status to his partner for fear of rejection and embarrassment and in some cases may not even know his own HIV status. Thus, they refer to this behavior as "negotiated danger" (Ekstrand et al. 1993). It seems then, much to many a gay man's, many an educator's, and many a researcher's displeasure, that even where there is agreement in the research concerning gay men and safer sex, there is also polarized disagreement; but so it is in a fuzzy world.

With the exception of ideological polarizations, some degree of disagreement is healthy and necessary. As disheartening as the situation may appear, without a degree of debate our understanding of sex, risky sex, sexual negotiation, and sexual decision-making would never advance, and dogma would replace inquiry. Unfortunately, though, these debates exist within an all-or-nothing heterodoxy where one perspective must be right and all others must be wrong.

It is into this contentious cauldron that my research and this book cautiously plunge, in an attempt to blur the culturally constructed theoretical battle lines by assuming that there may be multiple "correct" perspectives which may operate within differing circumstances. Put simply, all the research cited here may be accurate, but the applicability of the results to actual sexual practice depends upon the individual and his biological, sociocultural, and psychological being in relation to his sexual situations.

Pinpointing multiple sociocultural and psychological factors of import to sexual experience may occasion polite debate but will probably raise few disciplinary hackles. After all, in the spirit of fuzziness, qualitative researchers have often cautioned that sexual experience is shrouded in individual and social meanings that can only be understood by probing deeply into sex, sexual relationships, and specific sexual acts (Davis 1983; also see Gatter 1995). Insider and socially constructed meanings of unsafer sex are indeed weighty variables for ambiguous decisions, but they are only part of the picture. There is another, more disputatious and quarrelsome variable: biology. Even though the biology of sex is often ignored by HIV educators and researchers alike, human sexual arousal is also a neurophysiological event, not just a socially and psychologically constructed phenomenon, and this neurophysiology is grounded in humankind's evolutionary past.

Like any other group of people, gay men belong to the set of human animals, and like all humans, they are not perfect. Human beings have an evolutionary history of which sexual pleasure is a part. Along our evolutionary journey, we humans have acquired a desire or drive for sexual pleasure, and this desire or psychobiological drive evolved (or perhaps continued to evolve) during a time in which our ancestors were hunters and gatherers living in small groups and not plagued by sexually transmitted infectious agents (Abramson and Pinkerton 1995; Bailey and Aunger 1995; Harris 1979; Neese and Williams 1994). Furthermore, intertwined with this drive for pleasure there may well be an evolved need to escape boredom and to experience variety in our pleasure even if this pleasure is culturally or socially forbidden. "Humans tend to prefer a variety in all sensory modalities," argues Robert Edgerton, "and they find boredom so unpleasant that they frequently take dangerous risks to escape it" (1992:73).

It is under just such an overarching framework—one that takes into account the biological/evolutionary, sociocultural, and psychological explanations of amorphous human experience, sexual situations, the meaning of sex, and the role (or reduced role) of thought processes during sex—that I, with the testimonials of a diverse microcosm of gay men, will explore in the following chapters. The stories to come demonstrate the ambivalent nature of sexual practice and the inescapable failure that must ensue when one tries to affix neat or rigid predictors onto unpredictable individual sexual behaviors, situations, and decisions. From these specific yet singular accounts, I will attempt to transcend that sense of frustration and distress felt by educators and researchers who deplore the failure of gay men to comply totally with safer sex guidelines. These professionals have to realize that many gay men do in fact follow, at least some or most of the time, the recommendation to use a condom for anal sex.

However, we must also admit that we can expect to see the occasional risky sexual encounter, depending upon the situation and an individual's mental, physiological, and behavioral responses while performing in the heat of the moment (Bloor et al. 1992; Gold 1995; Gold et al. 1991).

But judge for yourself. Come meet the men of West Hollywood who are living, loving, and grieving, but still experiencing pleasure, beneath the dark eclipse of the century's most dangerous and deadly—but controllable—epidemic.

2

Johnny and Ralph: Commitment and Trust

The sleepers had all they needed. Only to lie like this between the bombs, dreaming away and not alone . . .

—Paul Monette, *Afterlife* (1990)

People always want some scandal beyond the scandal they're allowed.

—Diane Ackerman, *A Natural History of Love* (1994)

They kissed one another, and wept one with another, until David exceeded [himself].

And Jonathan said to David, Go in peace, forasmuch as we have sworn both of us in the name of the LORD, saying, The LORD be between me and thee, and between my seed and thy seed for ever.

—1 Samuel 20:41–42

Ralph telephoned me after he and Johnny had picked up one of my flyers at a West Hollywood coffee shop. The mint green announcement had called for gay men, aged thirty to forty-four, to participate in a study of gay male sexuality. As Ralph explained, "Both Johnny and I are gay, and we still have sex, believe it or not, after living together for eight years. We thought, why not?"

Although Johnny was much less enthusiastic than Ralph over the idea of spending a few hours talking about his sex life with an anthropologist, Ralph thought "it might be fun." In the end, Ralph won out and the couple made an appointment to meet at my home in West Hollywood. The day they arrived was one of those hot, smoggy days typical of a Southern California summer, a day certain to end in a spectacular sunset haze of yellow and red. It was a scorcher. But we made the most of the day, sipping on bottled water and chatting over the hum of the tape recorder and the soft whir of a rotating fan.

When I first met the couple at the door, I noticed right away a vis-
ible age difference between them. I soon found out that Johnny, the
reluctant one, was six years Ralph's senior. At thirty-nine, Johnny
had short, prematurely graying hair that was parted on the left and
combed with care. His face was mildly wrinkled from many years of
sunbathing whereas, in contrast, Ralph's face was clear, showing
none of the signs of a perpetual sun worshiper, and his lustrous
golden bangs brushed the top of his wire eyeglasses whenever he
shook his head.

Johnny appeared nervous. His hands trembled slightly and he
readily allowed Ralph to take the upper hand during our initial conversation. I feared Johnny might not stay for the interview, particularly after I informed them that I wanted to talk with each of them
separately rather than as a couple. Johnny's body language—ner-
vously glancing at the door or out a window while one leg shook
spasmodically—clearly communicated that he did not want to be
there. But he stayed.

I chose to interview Ralph first while Johnny waited out back in
my garden, under the shade of an old avocado tree. He later came
inside to watch television in the living room as I interviewed Ralph
in my back office. I hoped that this time would be sufficient for
Johnny to calm down and relax.

Ralph's interview was effortless on my part. He talked freely and
did not seem bothered by my probing personal questions. Johnny's
interview, on the other hand, commenced slowly. He initially responded to the interrogation with generally vague and short answers, a terse yes or no, but did not otherwise seem to mind my constantly asking him "what do you mean by that?" After we had
reviewed Johnny's childhood and his coming out as a gay man, he
became more animated and spoke with less restraint. The nervous
shaking that had plagued his right leg dissipated, and he appeared
to have mastered his uneasiness before we reached our discussion of
safer and unsafer sex. It was at that point that he related to me a
secretive experience. When I asked why he was willing to share
something so personal with me, indeed something that might wind
up in print, he responded, "That's what it's all about. Isn't it? I hope
my story can help others, and me as well."

Unlike the other case histories to come, instead of here dwelling upon Johnny and Ralph's childhoods, coming out stories, and individual experiences with AIDS, I will focus primarily on the time that Johnny and Ralph have spent together (eight years), starting with the day they first met and then began to fall in love.

The First Meeting

Johnny and Ralph met in a "neighborhood bar" in New York City's Greenwich Village on a fall evening in 1986. Johnny was visiting New York on business, and as he would "often" do, stayed over for a weekend of diversion and sex. New York gave him a reprieve from the "uptight" ambiance of the West Hollywood bar scene and the warm weather back home. Although he would "never even consider" leaving West Hollywood for good, he sometimes tired of the monotonous California sunshine and felt that a bit of cool weather, maybe even some rain, would be agreeable for a change. He told me that he had not "the teeniest inkling" that a fortuitous sexual meeting on this very weekend would change his life forever.

> JOHNNY: I always liked visiting New York, especially in the fall when the weather was cool and the leaves were turning. That's why I'd always jump at the chance to visit our clients there. I decided to stay over that weekend and go out to some of the bars in New York. I thought it would give me a break from the hot and sunny summer back home and I really needed a change of scene.
>
> I went to a neighborhood type bar in the Village and that was when I saw Ralph for the first time. He was cute and preppie, drinking a Heineken at the bar. I went over, struck up a conversation, and one thing led to another.
>
> RALPH: I had been shopping all day long that Saturday. I used to love to shop. I was pretty exhausted—shopping does wear one out—so I went to have a drink at my usual hangout. Well . . . I probably had about three or four before Johnny came over. I had been there for quite a while, unwinding. I wasn't looking to pick someone up that night. I just wanted to relax, have a few drinks, and then go home. I was truly exhausted.
>
> When Johnny came over it was a big, nice surprise. I remember that he sat down beside me. I thought at the time, "What a hunk." He was older, though he didn't have any gray hairs. He was wearing a parka.

I remember that because he looked like a conservative person, which I like. Someone who could easily pass for Mr. Cleaver on *Leave It to Beaver*. One of my activist friends insists that I am ashamed [of being gay] because I don't get into doing drag and the clone-ish look, and I like older, straight-looking types. It's not that I am ashamed of being gay. It's just that I like that [conservative] type of man. It's not that I'm looking for a father figure either. He [Johnny] wasn't like my father at all. My father was working class, a factory worker. I just find successful-looking men who are slightly older than me to be super sexy. I really don't know why.

The bar was smoky like it always was, but Johnny didn't smoke and that was a plus. I had just finished another beer and was getting a little bit tipsy. I noticed he kept looking over my way, and our eyes may have made contact a couple of times, but I was sort of shy and I'd always look down when a guy was looking at me. . . . I think he asked me if I wanted another beer and I did. We did sit and talk for a while. We laughed and talked a lot about current issues. It was nice to talk to someone who could talk about more than sex and money. He was clearly aware and intelligent and, like I said, definitely my type. That final beer must've loosened up my shyness because the next thing I knew I was inviting him to my apartment, which was a rare thing for me to do. Normally if I had sex, I'd go to the other guy's place.

The sex was great. It was very romantic and touchy. He definitely was the leader and he cuddled me all night. We talked a lot that night about all sorts of things and spent all of Sunday together walking around New York until he had to fly back to LA.

For approximately six months, Ralph and Johnny sustained a long-distance dating relationship, and they were falling in love. In March 1987, Ralph, frustrated by the geographical distance between them, pressured Johnny into making a definitive choice. Ralph wanted a monogamous relationship "modeled on" the infamous American television couple from the late 1950s and early 1960s, "the Cleavers," so he gave Johnny an ultimatum.

RALPH: Johnny was my dream relationship. It was almost like we could move to the suburbs, adopt a kid, and live happily ever after just like the Cleavers. He was successful and didn't have any problems with drugs and alcohol. That was important to me. I had dated a couple of guys who drank too much and it was a disaster. That sounds funny . . . you know . . . especially since I was sort of drunk on the night we met.

But I don't have a problem with alcohol. I can take it or leave it. Johnny and I had so much in common: music, taste in clothing, and other things. We'd go shopping together and always be drawn to the same furniture or clothes. Our sex life, when we were together, was very romantic. He always brought me flowers and doted so much attention on me. It was like a dream come true.

I was madly in love with Johnny as you can see, but our relationship could not continue as it was. We talked several times a week on the telephone and would spend time together when he was working in New York, but it got to be more and more difficult to say goodbye when he had to fly back to LA. Yes, I thought about going out with other people, but I couldn't. I was in love. Terribly so. I wanted a relationship, and so I took a chance and forced him to make a decision.

JOHNNY: Ralph called me at home one night. He sounded very moody and serious. He said he had something very important to tell me, and I thought, "Oh no. I hope it isn't serious like AIDS or something." I was relieved when it was about something else, something that had been on my mind too. He told me that either our relationship would have to end or one of us would move, and he was willing to make the move to LA. I was in love with Ralph too, but I had also been seeing a guy in West Hollywood off and on. It wasn't the same as with Ralph though. I just didn't connect with this other guy. Ralph and I have so much in common. We both like classical music. We like to go to the theater. We like the same type of furniture. Sometimes it was like we were always thinking the same things. It just felt right. He is such a great guy and he's intelligent. He can carry on a conversation, which most queens in West Hollywood can barely accomplish without lapsing into [a discussion about] the latest top 40 hit or something else incredibly stupid. When we met, he struck me as real, not a fake. He seemed honest. To make a long story short, Ralph moved in with me and got a job right away. He's a very together guy.

Monogamy, Sex, and Jealousy

Before they met and moved in together, Johnny, being older, had had more sexual experience than Ralph. In the late 1970s, prior to any awareness of HIV and its consequences, Johnny was delving into homosexual sex while Ralph did not begin to explore sex with men until 1984, just two years before he met Johnny and a time when AIDS awareness was just beginning to take a solid hold within the gay com-

munity. This decade-long gap in coming out colors each man's interpretation of and feelings about condoms and safer sex, and it was
when discussing the 1970s and his past that Johnny revealed more of
himself to me. His speech cadence quickened and was punctuated
with momentary pauses as he collected his thoughts.

> JOHNNY: In the 1970s I was kind of into the sex scene. I may look like
> your average conventional guy, but I still got around a lot. I went out
> virtually every single weekend possible, but I never got into the baths
> and such. . . . They weren't my style. I like to see what I am screwing,
> and I like to see a guy more than once, but I may have dated several
> guys at a time. It's more intimate that way [dating a guy more than
> once]. One-night stands were OK, especially after the fact, if I knew
> that it wasn't worth pursuing. . . . There were a lot of flaky ones back
> then: alcoholics, drug addicts, and guys wasting their lives looking for
> sex night and day. I've always preferred guys who at least seemed to
> have a head on their shoulders, and I wouldn't know that unless we at
> least had a conversation before, or sometimes—I'm afraid to admit
> it—after sex. When I dated a guy, I'd romance him with candy and
> flowers. . . . Sounds corny. I know that probably makes me different
> from some of the other guys you've interviewed. [*I shrug my shoulders,
> but I don't verbally respond*]
>
> I never liked disco music and the all-night dancing. I'm trained in
> the violin and like a different style of music, but I'd go along with it
> sometimes just so I could meet other gay guys. . . . In reality, I'm more
> down-to-earth. I wanted a relationship, but it was difficult back then
> to find a guy who would settle down and not party all the time. . . . I
> wanted someone with a life outside of gay sex, somebody I could
> spend a good part of my life with.
>
> Condoms weren't used at all back then. Never. AIDS wasn't around
> then. I got gonorrhea once, but other than that, not a lot [of sexually
> transmitted diseases] like other guys. I've always liked guys that are a
> little younger than me, and so I was mostly the top. I always found
> being the bottom [anal receptor] way too painful. I don't understand
> how it can be pleasurable, but it obviously is for some guys. . . . Thank
> goodness. . . . I guess that [being the top] helped keep me HIV nega-
> tive. I know you can get it [HIV] even if you're a top, but it's a little
> worse for the other guy, at least that's what I hear.
>
> Then in the 1980s, when the word started getting out about AIDS,
> people started getting sick and groups of gay men got into handing
> out condoms on the corner. So I started using condoms. . . . Not at

first, because we thought that those guys [handing out condoms] were overreacting, but with everybody dying, it didn't take long to catch on. . . . I was really afraid. I remember if I had a one-night stand, I would go home and shower and scrub. Like I thought, I guess, that soap and water might get rid of the AIDS thing that I imagined on my body. I used to look at every bruise like it might be cancer and was always relieved when it changed from purple to yellow or black. I later calmed down.

When Ralph and I met, we used condoms up until the time that he moved in with me, and then we stopped. . . . Sex feels so much better without a condom, and Ralph wanted me to ejaculate inside him. I didn't resist. It was great not to have to worry about a rubber. It was more romantic, and like I said it feels much better. Condoms were always a nuisance anyway, just something we had to do to keep from getting sick.

RALPH: I didn't have my first sexual experience with a man, other than fooling around a little with guys at school, until I left Missouri and moved to New York in 1983. I can't remember for sure. I think I was hesitant about having sex with guys, not because of homophobia— even though we were working class, my family was fairly liberal—but because I was afraid of getting AIDS. I was living in New York where a lot of gays were coming down with it. When I started out having sex, I always used condoms every single time. I'm what you'd call a bottom, and so it's somewhat more risky for me. I knew that and that's why I always insisted on a condom every time. Sometimes I can be a top, but it's not my preferred position. I can't believe I'm telling you this, but I guess this is what it's all about. . . .

One time, I was with a guy who didn't want to put one [a condom] on, so I told him to put it on or I would leave. Well he didn't, and I left. I felt like crap afterwards, but I'm glad I didn't let him do it to me without one. That would have been stupid. I couldn't understand why this guy would even dare to try and do that. I just can't understand it. Guys who have sex without a condom must be suicidal or have a death wish or something. I don't get it. . . .

I didn't have sex with lots of guys before I met Johnny. I had a few one-nighters here and there, but not a lot. I dated a couple of guys for two or three months each, but the relationships sort of wilted. I was looking for a true monogamous relationship. I was in love with being in love, more than I was interested in having lots of sex. Then along came Johnny and he whisked me away. I was very excited by it all. It took so much energy trying to find the right man.

After I moved to LA, we stopped using condoms. Before Johnny, I never knew what sex without a condom felt like. I think it was my idea to stop using them. Maybe. I'm not sure. But whoever brought it up, the other one didn't refuse. Sex without a condom feels a hell of a lot better. I mean a lot. It's like the difference between a bicycle and a stretch limo. It might just be in my head, but having sex without a condom means a lot to me, especially with Johnny.

Having sex without a condom is for Ralph more than physical pleasure. As I noted in chapter 1, anal sex without condoms for couples is loaded with meaning, including a signification of trust and commitment.

RALPH: I like to have Johnny ejaculate inside of me because it brings us closer together. If he didn't, it would seem like something—I don't know what—would be missing. It's as important to me as an orgasm. It's difficult to explain, but it means that he is mine and I am his. It's just him and me, together as one. I don't know why heterosexuals can't understand that. I'm sure a woman feels the same way when her husband ejaculates inside her. I don't think it's any different with heterosexual couples. It means a union. Cumming together at the same time, with him inside me. It's almost a spiritual thing. Of course it feels physically good too, and that's very important, but it's love. It's a spiritual joining of our bodies, like being one. Ooh, I got shivers just thinking about it. Oh my . . . [*He fans his face with his right hand*]

Anyway, moving on, I trusted Johnny completely and we got rid of the condoms pretty darn quick, even though neither of us knew our HIV status. We thought that we both probably had it [AIDS]. We didn't get tested until 1987, and we went together for the test and to get our results. We were both so worried, but luckily, we both turned out to be negative. Thank God! I remember we went out to dinner, drank at least two bottles of champagne, and made jokes about getting hit by a car on the way home. You know, like we didn't get AIDS, but we'd get killed the old-fashioned way like being run down by a careless driver, and after all that worrying about our test results. It sounds sick, but I think we were coming down from all that tension while waiting to find out. After that, we promised each other to be true to one another and not to have sex with other people. Neither of us had cheated on each other, or at least I hadn't.

As can be expected in any relationship, Johnny and Ralph have had their moments of crisis. According to Johnny, their first "real" argument revolved around Johnny's reluctance and ultimate refusal to come out as gay to his parents.

JOHNNY: Oh yes, I remember our first fight. It was a real doozie—in 1988. My parents were passing through LA and were going to spend a few days at our place. I've never told my parents that I am gay. . . . I always feel like, well, why rock the boat? I get along just fine with them. . . . They're very conservative, and I think they'd have a difficult time coming to grips with my sexuality. I wanted to get the place ready and make it look like Ralph and I were just roommates instead of lovers. Set up a separate bedroom. Put away anything around the house that might be obviously gay.

Ralph went crazy on me. He screamed and yelled and said so many nasty things to me. I mean really nasty, like calling me a sick, self-loathing faggot or something close to that. He left and stayed at a friend's house during my parents' entire visit. He said something to the effect that he didn't want to be a part of my cover-up. He was really pissed—I'd never seen him so angry—so he left for a few days. It was a pretty miserable visit with my parents. I missed Ralph and I felt like a shit.

He came home as soon as my parents were out and on their way. He said he was sorry, but I pouted for days—I guess to make him feel bad for treating me the way he did. But we made up and I was very apologetic for trying to hide our relationship. I told him that if my parents ever visited again, I would tell them, but I've never had to follow through with it. They have never visited. I'd hate to have to do it.

Ralph's memory of their first argument deviates from that of Johnny's. Instead of an argument about coming out, Ralph recalls that it involved jealousy.

RALPH: We had been living together less than a year. I used to be terribly jealous when I was younger. One of Johnny's old flames rang him up once and left a message on our machine, and Johnny called him back. They talked for a little while, but I don't remember what about. I couldn't hear everything Johnny was saying, but I know they made a date to go out to lunch a few days later. That was the day I followed Johnny. I'm not kidding you. It sounds ridiculous, but I told you I was jealous. I can't believe that I was so immature.

While Johnny and his friend were eating, I was sitting not more than, say, three or four tables away, and of course Johnny saw me. He completely ignored me and started flirting with the other guy. Touching him across the table. Smiling a lot. That sort of thing. He really tried to set me off and get back at me for following him. His little revenge worked really well, and I was absolutely furious. I left the restaurant virtually in tears and rushed home. When Johnny arrived home about an hour or so later, he didn't say a word to me about what had happened. He was giving me the cold treatment and I got even more ticked off. Really PO'ed. When I finally let out my anger, it was terribly spiteful. I called him everything I could think of that was not civil. I told him to go and fuck the guy if that was what he wanted to do. So Johnny left very angry. Then I felt like crap.

I waited and waited for him to come home. He finally did about four or five hours later. Drunker than a skunk too. I really wanted to make up. I felt like a silly little schoolgirl. I told him I was sorry, and then I guess it was his turn to lash out at me. He let me have it [not physically but with words]. In retrospect, it was all very childish of me. Our relationship has matured since then. We finally made up the next day and had the most wonderful sex. I never, ever, followed him again. I wanted to trust him, and as difficult as it was, I didn't pull another stunt like that one again.

Both Johnny and Ralph described Ralph as the more jealous partner, but Johnny was quick, at least initially, to downplay Ralph's jealousy. On the other hand, Ralph laid out his "good reasons" for possessing vigilant suspicions.

JOHNNY: Ralph is less jealous than he used to be, but he is still highly suspicious. He usually wants to know who I'm talking to on the phone, who I am going to lunch with, where I'm going, and that sort of thing. If I mention the name of a guy he doesn't recognize, he gives me the third degree. But he doesn't interfere with my cruising anymore like he used to do. . . . It [cruising] is not really sexual. . . . It's not that I would do anything with guys who cruise me, but it's sort of good for my self-esteem to be in the Mayfair [a West Hollywood grocery store] and to cruise a guy on the other side of the oranges or next to the broccoli. Even though I'm in a relationship and getting older, it makes me feel good when other guys find me attractive. . . . It's sort of sad, but it tells me that I've still got what it takes to attract other men.

Up until the last couple of years, Ralph would always nudge me and make snide comments when he'd catch me cruising, like "would you look at the real fruit?" One time he walked right between me and the other guy and then looked at me, then at him, and shook his head like he was disgusted. It was always such a scene. . . . He used to be very insecure, but he's much better now.

RALPH: I rarely so much as look at another guy, but Johnny is always cruising. It still bothers me, but I don't make such a big deal about it anymore. I am very jealous, but not without my reasons. Johnny has slept around on me. I am sure of it. He told me about one of his affairs, but I didn't want to hear any of the details. Other than that one, I hope he hasn't slept with other guys, but I am pretty sure he has. I'm not sure how I know this, but I just feel it. He travels a lot for his job, and if I call his room pretty late, he sometimes isn't there. He always makes excuses, like he was down at the hotel bar or having a meeting with a straight client, but I never know for sure. I love him, but I don't truly trust him sexually. I sometimes think with his cruising that he wants to flaunt it in my face, but I guess I'm a little hypersensitive. I always tell myself that he loves me. He really does.

Even though he suspects Johnny's infidelity, Ralph will not approach the topic of condoms within the relationship, partly for fear of discovery that his suspicions about Johnny's sexual trysts might in reality be more than just his mental concoctions. Moreover, although he is skeptical about Johnny's sexual commitment, Ralph trusts him not to put their lives at risk.

RALPH: If he does sleep around, I hope he uses a condom. I'm sure he does. He's ultra-responsible. There's no way I'd talk to him about using a condom when we make love, because he would think that I was accusing him of having sex with other men, and like I said, I'm not sure if he has done it more than that one time I mentioned earlier. If he has done it with other men, I'm sure he would wear a condom. He's very aware and I know he would not put me or himself at risk for AIDS. He cares too much about me and about himself to do that. He loves me even if he may have slept around a few times.

The last two passages from Ralph opened up a Pandora's box for the rest of Ralph's and for most of Johnny's interview. First, I was curious about Johnny's side of the story concerning his alleged affair, and second, if Johnny was truly having sex outside the relationship, I wanted to inquire as to why the couple maintained at least the appearance of monogamy. Third, and perhaps most pressing to the issue at hand, I had to find out if Johnny used condoms during sex with other men, outside of his relationship with Ralph. I thought the answer to my first query might be difficult to unveil but, once told, the remaining information would surely follow.

Johnny was hesitant when I asked him, "Have you ever had sex outside of your relationship with Ralph?" I did not give a clue, at least that I am aware of, as to whether Ralph had disclosed one of Johnny's known affairs in his interviews, but Johnny probably suspected that Ralph would tell me. He began slowly, wavering a bit, but he composed himself as I leaned in to hear his version.

JOHNNY: Gosh, this is embarrassing. [*His face is pink*] I'm sure Ralph told you. Didn't he? [*I don't respond*] It was about a year ago. I told Ralph about it. I'm sure he told you. . . . [*Again, I don't respond*] Ralph went to visit his folks for a couple of days, but I couldn't get away from work. We hadn't had sex with each other for a couple of weeks, and as I've already told you, I'm more sexual than he is. He would settle for sex once a week. That'd be enough for him. Once a week. Not me.

I went down to the Different Light [a gay bookstore] and flipped through the men's magazines [pornography] on the rack in the back of the store. You probably know that it's pretty cruisy back there. [*I nod*] I thought I would buy a couple of those magazines to take care of my horniness. Masturbation material. There was a young-ish guy, probably twenty-something, flipping through one of the magazines and standing pretty close to me. I could feel that he was glancing up at me between the pages, and I was getting turned on by his cruising me. . . . He wasn't great looking, just average, but like I said I was fairly horny, and I like it when younger guys cruise me. . . . It makes me feel good. I bought one of the magazines and started to walk home. I noticed he was looking at me when I left, and sure enough, I turned around and could see that he was following me. I stopped and sort of shuffled my feet a little, looking at the ground. I was a little nervous. He came up and said something about the magazine that I'd bought. I don't remember exactly what. We talked a little bit, exchanged names, and I brought him over to my place. That was all. . . . It was just a release. I didn't care about the guy. . . . It wasn't like when I was single and wanted to get to know the guy. And it was safe. He had a condom with him and I used it to screw him. It wasn't dangerous at all . . . but I still felt guilty about it.

I told Ralph about it during one of his interrogations. I couldn't stand his accusing me anymore. . . . So I just thought, "to hell with it," and I told him the truth. He didn't want to hear about it and threatened to move out. He didn't speak to me for a week or so, but we eventually made up after I promised him that it would never happen again.

Despite Johnny's infidelity, the couple considers their relationship to be a monogamous one. Monogamy is of the utmost importance to Ralph, but Johnny struggles to suppress private desires for a non-monogamous sexual agreement.

RALPH: Monogamy is very important to me. It's a commitment. I know Johnny loves me and wants a monogamous relationship, but unfortunately, he is a man and men have hyper sex drives. I swear it. It has got to be genetic or something. I mean, look at lesbians. They don't sleep around so much like gay men do. Not that Johnny sleeps around a lot. I just mean that I only know for sure about that one time. I want us to grow old together. I can't imagine it any other way. I will always love him and I know that he will always love me. . . .

Don't get me wrong. I'm no Doris Day. I look at guys too, but I'm not as blatant about it as he is. I may have fantasies about other men— and I don't think there's anything wrong with that. It's probably healthy. But I only have sex, exclusively, with Johnny. I've never cheated on him, and I couldn't imagine really sleeping with another guy. I just couldn't. When he's out of town, I'll rent porno and jerk off, but I wouldn't dream of having sex with someone else. It's important to me to maintain my commitment.

I know some guys who have open relationships, but I don't think they really work. I don't know any open relationship that has survived time. Besides, I like having only one guy to hold, kiss, and care for. I can't imagine the energy it would take to juggle more than one guy, and I would really be jealous if there was another guy to compete with, not only in a sexual way but for attention and emotional attachment too.

Still, it is just such an open relationship that Johnny would prefer, a relationship that would allow him to have novel sexual liaisons with other men, but nonetheless one that is bounded by mutually agreed upon rules. Rules are common in open relationships between gay men. A negotiated code of behavior may include "rules about information and honesty, rules about regularity and emotional distance, rules about discretion and politeness, rules about threesomes, and rules about safer sex" (Davies et al. 1993).

In regard to an open relationship, Johnny singled out two of the above regulations to be of importance to him. His archetypal relationship would include rules about emotional distance (i.e., not falling in love with another man) and rules about discretion and politeness (i.e., not flaunting it in front of Ralph or friends and acquaintances). Noticeably missing from Johnny's regulations, however, are rules about safer sex.

In spite of his desire for a relationship of a different sort, Johnny keeps this idea to himself and does not share it with Ralph for fear of losing him.

> JOHNNY: Ideally, I'd like an open relationship, one in which I can go out and have sex with other men on occasion—not often, just every now and then. I like sex a lot, a lot more than Ralph likes it. . . . Sometimes I just want to try something new, explore a new body, something different. Don't misunderstand me. I love Ralph more than I have ever loved anyone. Anyone. I really mean that. We do a lot of different things together sexually, but it's not the same as touching an unknown body, one that you don't touch all the time. . . .
>
> If we had an open relationship, there would be rules. We would have to be discreet, not throw it in each other's faces, and not be seen around with another man in front of other people we know. . . . I guess I can be just as jealous as Ralph. So it would have to be for sex only and absolutely no dating. That would be threatening. Sex is one thing, but dating and love are another.
>
> I can never let Ralph know this. He has his mind set on monogamy and it's very, very important to him. . . . I guess that is what relationships are about: you have to give and take. Besides, the person I am in a relationship with is more important than the type of relationship. I'll make this sacrifice for Ralph.

Negotiated Risk

Ralph and Johnny's relationship posits the essence of the debate between proponents of negotiated danger versus backers of negotiated safety. As I noted in chapter 1, the debate between the two perceptions of risk hinges upon whether honesty and trust exist in the relationship and whether HIV status is truly known by both partners.

For now, Ralph and Johnny know that they are both HIV negative. Thus far I have presented one case of Johnny's infidelity, and he is adamant about its having been a safer encounter. Therefore, on the surface, it would appear that they fit the negotiated safety model. However, on the negotiated danger side, there is a lack of trust and honesty between them. Johnny has not been entirely truthful with Ralph about his sexual urges and desires. But what really is of utmost concern here is whether this absence of trust and honesty translates into risk for HIV infection, which would only be the case if Johnny or Ralph had or is having unprotected sex with other men. As the interview progressed, Johnny disclosed one such case.

> JOHNNY: Yes, there were other times that I have cheated on Ralph, but only a couple. They were . . . well, . . . one of them was not safe. See. I said it. . . . [*He pauses and leans forward*] It was eight months ago in New York when I was traveling. . . . [*He leans back into his chair*] I picked this guy up at a club and brought him back to my hotel room. . . . Neither of us had any condoms. I'd had a few drinks and he was sort of smashed. . . . [*I ask him why they didn't just have oral sex or masturbate together*] Good question. I don't know. It was all so sudden-like. Initially that was all I was intending to do. . . . We didn't talk about it before we got started. I just assumed that he intended to have safer sex too. We were making out and he was doing me orally. I reached over to feel his behind. He was very young, maybe twenty-five or so and cute too. All of a sudden he stopped, rolled over onto his stomach, stuck his butt in the air, and waited. And I did it [penetrated his anus]. . . . I didn't think about it. I had forgotten about condoms. The sex, the hotel, and all of it. I was really worked up by the thrill of the cheat. But I just did it. I pulled out before I ejaculated. I'd asked him his HIV status before we even got started, because of the oral sex. . . . He said he was negative.

It appears, then, that there is some risk involved in Ralph and Johnny's case, but the risk is more one of degree and does not fit neatly within either of the two extreme categories of "negotiated safety" and "negotiated danger." Many variables are involved in determining the degree of risk involved for both Ralph and Johnny. Thus instead of applying labels such as safety or danger, perhaps a less definite, more fluid and flexible terminology is needed. I prefer the term *negotiated risk*. Negotiated risk allows for diverse situations.

For example, if Johnny's young sexual partner was truly HIV negative when they were having sex, then there is no cause for concern. If he was HIV positive but believed he was negative because he had not been tested recently, then the risk may be of consequence. The risk of infection for Ralph may also be increased or decreased depending upon the type of sexual acts he practiced with Johnny following Johnny's "cheat" as well as upon Johnny's later testing behavior—that is, if Johnny continues to be tested and can confirm his HIV-negative status. If Ralph and Johnny only practiced oral sex, for instance, until Johnny got another accurate HIV-negative antibody test, then there is still little risk. On the other hand, risk would be increased if Johnny forwent testing and did not confirm that he had been spared infection. Fortunately for Ralph, his risk was somewhat reduced by Johnny's testing and sexual actions following his moment of pleasure.

> JOHNNY: I never told Ralph. We weren't having a lot of sex at the time, and so for the first few months after that night, I avoided sex [with Ralph]. I made excuses like being too tired and not feeling very well. We only had anal sex once during that time without a condom and I faked orgasm. . . . I didn't want to come inside of him. . . . I felt so ashamed and couldn't understand why I would take such a risk, a risk that would jeopardize my life, Ralph's life, and my relationship with him. Then about three months ago [five months following possible exposure], I got my test results. They were negative and I had been really sweating it out. I'll never ever do that again. It wasn't worth it to me. . . . I worried so much about it. I was mostly worried for Ralph. At least I got a moment's pleasure out of it. . . . I know the guy told me he was HIV negative, but you never really know. If he had unsafe sex with me . . . well, . . . then he's probably done the same with others, maybe even after his last test. . . .
>
> There were times when I would start to tell him [Ralph]. I'd look across the room or the table and he'd be busy doing whatever, reading or watching television. I wanted to tell him. . . . But I couldn't get the words to come out. I just couldn't. . . . He'd have freaked out. Completely freaked, and so I've kept it to myself. . . . I am such a coward. Aren't I? [*I don't respond*]

The Future

The lack of honesty and trust between these two men, a vacuum which could have a cataclysmic result, is lamentable but, notwithstanding their predicament, Ralph and Johnny were both resolute in their belief that they will be together as time progresses and they reach their years of senescence.

> RALPH: We'll be together for years to come. I know that with all my heart. We have so much in common and share the same goals in life. We are best friends and share most everything. There are times when I look at him and it's as if we were meeting for the first time. We are affectionate with each other and take time to listen. I'll ask him about his day and he'll ask about mine. We're interested in each other's activities.
>
> I'm working on my jealousy and I'm trying to put more trust in Johnny. He is the best thing that has ever happened to me. If it were to end, I'm sure I'd fall in love again, but this is different and there could never be a replacement. He really is a wonderful, loving man.
>
> JOHNNY: I know that I'll never make the same mistake again by doing something as stupid as having sex with a stranger without a condom. I love Ralph so much that if he wants a monogamous relationship, I'll work at it. We've started therapy and I hope this will help us work things out. My only fear is that I will have to be totally honest with Ralph and come clean about my fooling around. My therapist said that it will not work unless I am honest. . . . So, . . . I know I'll have to tell him [Ralph]. Maybe he'll try to understand. . . . Disclosure is not easy for me. Like I haven't come out to my parents or people at work. I wish I had more courage.
>
> Ralph is working on his jealousy and I'll work on my philandering. It's a two-way street and we're both dedicated to this relationship and to each other. I'm not getting any younger and I hope—no, I know—that he will be there for me. I love him so much. . . . I know this sounds like a trite Hallmark card, but he truly is very special to me.

So special that Johnny cannot be candid about his secretive sex life for fear of sacrificing his relationship. But he was relieved to finally be able to tell someone his secret. Just before the interview ended, Johnny sighed with apparent contentment. "Share my story," he urged more than once. "Maybe it'll prevent somebody else from doing something as stupid as I did. Life is too valuable and it is love that makes life livable." When we joined Ralph in the living room, Johnny embraced him, and as the couple shuffled to the front door, Johnny's right hand traced Ralph's lower back as if he had something he wanted to say.

3 Bob: Oral Pleasures

Pretty boys, beautiful men still swim in their pleasure like dolphins . . .

—Richard Harteis, "The Dolphins" (1989)

Like other human beings, I desire the experience. I want to hold this man and kiss him. Is this wanting too much? . . . Can any straight person understand what it is like to want to make love but to be terrified that to do so means possible death?

—Larry Kramer, *Reports from the Holocaust* (1989)

I interviewed thirty-four-year-old Bob at my home in April 1994. It was a sunny day, but a cool breeze stirred and permitted us to comfortably sip coffee at my kitchen table. Bob appeared to be a very serious man. While brushing back his military haircut, as if he had recently worn a longer, fuller style of his slate-black hair, he leaned his athletic shoulders forward and aimed his intense dark eyes directly at me from across the table. He rarely lowered his eyes, and it almost seemed as if he were going to interview me. I must admit that I was more than a little disconcerted at first.

Bob was eager to participate in the study and to tell his story. He would lightly pound his fist on the table from time to time in order to emphasize a point. The heavy French roast coffee accelerated his speech, allowing an occasional slip into his natural southern drawl as he became increasingly talkative, sharing his coming out process, his difficulties in maintaining relationships, and his oral pleasures. Unfortunately, his eagerness left few openings for me to dwell upon any given topic, as his train of thought appeared to jump ahead his ability to speak.

Childhood

Bob is one of three children born into a "prominent" and "respected" family that resided in a small town in western Oklahoma where his European ancestors had settled more than one hundred and fifty years ago. At the age of six, before Bob entered first grade, his father accepted a job in New York, and his family relocated . The move from a small town to a large city was a significant event for Bob as it laid open to him an unfamiliar world of new opportunities. It gave him the option of assuming a fresh and less restricted community role with greater anonymity.

> My mom is from New York and she kind of forced my dad to move up to New York and to take on this opportunity up there. Moving to New York was a big thing for me. It got me out of Oklahoma. I might still be there today if we hadn't moved. The schools were much better [in New York]. . . . It was great because I was no longer somebody because of my family's last name. . . . I mean . . . because of my last name, I had a lot to live up to in Oklahoma. I had to behave a certain way, and only play with certain acceptable children. Whereas in New York I could just start over and define myself however I wanted to be.

Five years after his arrival in New York, Bob temporarily returned to Oklahoma. When he was around eleven years old, Bob's parents divorced. Subsequent to that milestone event in his life history, his mother bought a cattle ranch and took Bob and his two siblings back with her to Oklahoma. Although during this period Bob traveled back and forth between New York and Oklahoma, within a year he returned to New York to live permanently with his father, but his brother and sister remained behind with their mother. Bob speaks a great deal about his father and, contrary to the experiences of numerous other gay men (Herdt 1989), as a child he sensed a closeness to his father that was much stronger than the slightly more distant relationship that he possessed with his mother.

> My mom was a real cattle person and my dad was allergic to them. I became allergic too, so I couldn't live full time with my mom, my brother, and my sister because during the summers they were going to all these cattle shows and state fairs. I couldn't do that. . . . So . . . you know . . . I had to spend a lot of time at home by myself. I went back to live with my dad. Then at least I wasn't at home alone all the time, and I was closer to my dad.

I couldn't believe my parents stayed together as long as they did, because they were never really in love. I think they thought they would grow to be in love, which is not a good way to start a marriage. My dad was from a prominent family, and there were a lot of people putting pressure on him to get married. His younger brother was married and already had a kid. And in that small town, living with your parents and being in your thirties like my father, people got real suspicious [of his sexuality]. He felt a lot of pressure to get married.

One day he saw my mother's picture in a college newspaper and called her to ask her out. She refused, but he was persistent.

They're very different people. My mother is very passionate, very emotional. My father suppresses all his feelings and avoids controversy. My mother would do things like buy furniture just to try and make my father mad. They never really communicated.

My father was a wonderful man and was always under pressure. He always wanted to be a lawyer, but his father demanded that he go to college and come back and work at the family business. He did what his father wanted and resented it for the rest of his life. He resented being dictated to all the time and not having a lot of choices. I guess that's why he went to the other extreme with his kids. He would never tell us what to do, and it was difficult to get direction from him. But I was close to him.

Before moving back to New York, that year in Oklahoma had a considerable impact on Bob's sexuality, in particular on his capacity to manage the stigma associated with being gay in heterosexual settings (see Plummer 1978).

I think I probably got better at hiding my sexuality because I had this experience going back and forth between Oklahoma and New York, between two different families really. I was never totally open. I could sort of be one person in one place and another person in the other place. That contributed to my adult life. You know, I have a go-go gay life, and I have my corporate life or whatever. Each is compartmentalized.

Around the age of six, Bob had already realized that he was attracted to the same sex; remembrance of same-sex attraction at such a young age is not unusual for gay men (Herdt 1992). But Bob did not have what he considered to be a "real" sexual experience until he was eleven years old. In retrospect, real sex for Bob means that, for the first time, he experienced penetration (oral) and he took this carnal experience to be more than a childhood game.

When he was a member of a local cub scout troop, Bob "fooled around" with other boys before he had "real sex." Fooling around included masturbation, touching each other's penises, and humping in imitation of sexual intercourse. In contrast, during and after his first "real" sexual experience, he felt a warm attachment beyond friendship, and for the first time he acknowledged to himself that it was not improbable, nor inherently bad, for him to care emotionally for another male.

> Ever since I was a kid at about six years old or so, I found myself attracted to men in a way that was too much for me to even think about. I was too young to have sex, but when I was in the fifth grade [ten years old], I had to go to gym class and change into gym clothes in the boy's locker room. I had like this raging hard-on. I didn't really know what it was. I just knew that I wasn't supposed to have one. When I was in cub scouts and boy scouts, I remember fooling around with boys, masturbating each other and sometimes laying on top of each other naked and rubbing our penises together.
>
> But later I had sex for the first time with a friend from school. We were sort of sleeping together in junior high school. With him, that was the first time that I ever put a penis inside my mouth or inside me at all. It was the first time that I had ever understood anything about sexuality, and I fell in love for the first time. I remember feeling sort of warm—you know. . . . Sounds corny . . . but, oh well. It was a very healthy relationship for two people being so young. I guess you'd call it a relationship. We were both popular with other kids. He was very talented. He could write poetry, and he could compose music. He was also an athlete. He sort of showed me that it was possible to be gay and a good person at the same time. I started to understand why I felt different from other boys. The thing he really did was teach me self-acceptance. He was comfortable with having sex with other boys, and in a small town that's very important. I didn't tell anyone.

Bob did not declare his new love and desire for other males to anyone. He concealed his newly found boyhood pleasures from his friends and from his entire family, including his brother (two years his senior and, it turned out, also gay). As often occurs with gay and lesbian youth, he did not associate his sexual behaviors with an identity, and he eventually experimented with heterosexuality (see Herdt 1992). "I didn't accept being gay yet, but I did accept that it was okay to have real sex with other boys. After my relationship with this guy,

I didn't really have a significant relationship with another guy. I dated women in the meantime and occasionally had sex with other boys. I still didn't know that I was gay."

Coming Out

For Bob, being "out" means both declaring his identity to others and developing his own sense of comfort with himself and his gay identity. Coming out is not a distinct event for him, but instead is a transformational process, a process which he is still undergoing (see Herdt 1992). There are milestones in this process though, such as frequenting gay bars and having sex with gay-identified men. He refers to these events as "living the gay life." As an adult, Bob is neither "completely out" nor "not out" but instead his "out-ness," if you will, is fuzzy, situational, and fluid through time and space (Cain 1991).

> I think coming out is a process. I don't know that there's a point in time that I became comfortable with being gay. I don't know that I'm totally comfortable with it today, but I'm certainly more comfortable with it today than I was ten years ago. I think I really pushed the accelerator on coming out when I got out of college. While I was in college, I spent a year in Europe and lived a gay life like going to gay clubs and screwing around with men. But then when I graduated, I moved out here [West Hollywood] and hit the gay bars. At least in my mind I was sort of out because I was living a gay life. I had gay friends. I was having gay sex. Although again, it was compartmentalized. I had my work life and then I had my gay life. Lately now, I've been much more open with people at work, but I don't see it [not being out at work] as a negative thing. . . .
>
> When I was in college, I was going to see this counselor because I was really unhappy about my sexuality. The one thing he said to me was, "Can you imagine what you'd be like if you weren't gay?" and I thought about it. I thought, "OK, if I weren't gay what would I be like?" I realized at that point that being gay was such an important part of me that I would be a completely different person if I weren't gay. I would have different motivations, completely different. [The counselor] really helped me. I have to remind myself sometimes that I am happy with myself and I accept myself. Once I realized that it wasn't something I could or would want to change, that was helpful for

me. I am still not completely out with everybody, you know. I still feel like a part of me just won't accept it, but I'm much further along.

Part of Bob's ongoing struggle to accept himself mirrors his parents' discordant coping reactions to Bob's disclosure of his being gay. Although Bob was closer to his father as a child, his divulgence of his sexuality and identity have limited communication between them. In contrast, disclosure has improved his relationship with his mother. By taking part in Bob's "gay life," his mother is seeking to understand him while striving to be an active participant in his world.

> My father is a very nice man, a kind man, but I can't talk about hard issues with him. When I talk about my sexuality, he gets real uncomfortable. He changes the subject. He literally will change the conversation in mid-sentence. Or I'll call him on the phone and I'll be telling him stories—something really important going on in my life—and he'll stop me in mid-sentence and say, "Well there's someone else that wants to say hello to you here." So he's really good with avoidance.
>
> Today my dad doesn't try hard enough, but my mother almost tries too hard. I'm still trying to educate them both. My mom can talk about it [Bob's being gay]. She's been to several gay bars. When she buys me a present, she's like "Oh honey, you'll like it. I got it in a gay store." She cried because she didn't go to the March on Washington [a massive political demonstration for gay rights in April 1993]. She watched it on TV in tears, and she said, "Next time I'm going to go. I'm going to march with the parents." She really tries to get involved and be a part of both my and my brother's lives.

Sex and Relationships Before AIDS

During the late 1970s Bob went to Europe, and it was there that he began his adult sexual exploration. AIDS was not yet prowling the corners of Bob's consciousness, and sex—both anal and oral penetration—was something to enjoy as he became slightly more "comfortable" with being a gay-identified man and as he lavished in the recreational side of sex.

> In Europe, I was just a little bit more comfortable with my sexuality and ready to play the field. It's not that I really had any relationships. I probably had sex a dozen times or something, but I was trying things out: I fucked and got fucked, sucked and got sucked . . . sometimes all

in one night. Nothing too kinky though. I'm not that adventurous. I went to these clubs where there were lots of gay men, and —wow!— there were so many possibilities. I think I was just realizing for the first time how much fun sex with another man can be when there are no strings attached.

Bob returned to the United States in 1980. Between 1980 and 1982, Bob's sex life was "very dry and there wasn't much happening." After he finished college in 1982, he moved to West Hollywood where he says "things picked up" as he forged a social network and formed enduring friendships by way of sex.

Then in 1982 I graduated from college and came to West Hollywood. I really hit the bars. I was going out every night, hoping to pick up a boy. I like them my age more or less. Then I met this boy who I had a relationship with for like a month. I was so happy. It was somebody that I really liked and he really liked me. But that didn't work out. I found out later that he usually had four-week relationships with people that he dated. Then I hooked up with these gay friends. Many of them I had had sex with, and unfortunately many of them are also dead today; but I really started making a life with a family of friends. That was great. We were young and free and comfortable with our sexuality. Going out. Having sex, sex, sex!

I finally dated someone for nine months straight . . . this guy named Joe. He was a nice guy, and really cute. Then I went to business school in the Northeast in 1984. So I left. December of that year after I had left, I found out that Joe had AIDS. This was 1984, and so like nobody knew [what to do about AIDS]. Nobody talked about condoms and safe sex. We used to have all kinds of unsafe sex. I fucked him and he fucked me. It's incredible to believe that Joe died.

Sex and Relationships After AIDS

Joe's illness jolted Bob into a panic. He became alarmed and apprehensive. For a short while, he avoided any and all sex, but his bid at practicing abstinence would not endure. Although he was not using condoms, he formed a "fuck buddy" relationship. (A fuck buddy is a steady partner for sex but is not necessarily a lover or a live-in relationship.) Bob thought that by having sex with just one person, he had reduced his risk for HIV transmission.

Looking back, Bob could not remember if his resolve to avoid sex, followed by "fuck buddy" monogamy, was self-induced or if it was influenced by the health education messages of the time which promoted partner reduction and abstinence. Nevertheless, Bob was ignorant of his and his fuck buddy's HIV status, and his strategy to reduce risk might have actually increased his risk if his partner had been HIV positive (Martin 1986), but in this case Bob believes he was "lucky." His fuck buddy was HIV negative.

> When Joe died, I went through this tremendous fear at school. He was dying and I was freaking out. I almost dropped out of school. I finally—I don't know how—made it through. I avoided sex. I was so afraid of it, and I associated it with death. But I couldn't go on forever like that, and I needed a release beyond masturbation. I wanted to play with another guy. Feel him. Smell him. I met this guy in business school and we were really like fuck buddies. We slept together a lot, and the sex was good. He's still a good friend of mine. Back in those days we still weren't getting the message yet, and we fucked a lot without condoms. I guess we may have heard this and that, but it's hard to remember if we weren't listening or if they [health educators] weren't talking. Then in 1985, Rock Hudson got sick. It hit the newspapers, and then I really freaked out. I quit having sex again altogether. That was how afraid I was.

Bob's fear and anxiety rose to the point that he adopted "drastic measures." He literally took flight from AIDS, landing a job based in London that required world travel. He clung to the notion that this move would minimize his chances of HIV infection.

> During this time, you know, the news was like AIDS was just in San Francisco, New York, and Los Angeles. Sometimes I heard it was in Africa. I was so afraid of the AIDS thing that I took a job in London and traveled all over the world for the next couple of years. I thought I would be safer outside of the United States. I was having a good bit of sex, at least once a week, but I was working long days and traveling around a lot.

While traveling abroad, Bob began to use condoms for anal sex. His adoption of condoms occurred not only in response to education and his experiences with AIDS (Gold 1993) but was also spawned by a medical doctor's warning.

I think I started using condoms at this time. It was interesting because when I was in Australia at one point—this is like in '87—they had these messages on TV. They had the grim reaper bowling down a group of ten people with a caption, "AIDS. It can strike anyone." So it really wasn't a safer sex message like "use a condom." It was fear-based advertising and not at all what I needed. But when I was in England, they sent out a pamphlet to every home telling what AIDS is and how you can get it. I don't remember the message. I just remember thinking, "God. Thank goodness I'm here. It's so much worse in the States."

I think it was my doctor who told me the real scoop on condoms. He said, "You know, if you use condoms, you won't get it [HIV]." Pretty much he told me that HIV was hard to get and if you use condoms you can prevent it [infection], so I started using condoms for anal sex. It was a good thing too, especially when I came back again [to West Hollywood]. I liked traveling around a lot, but I decided to move back to the West Hollywood area around 1990 because so many of my friends were sick and dying.

Before his return to the States, Bob was smitten by another American living in Australia. Although Bob was exceedingly attracted to this man, at first Bob and his new "love" practiced only safer sex. Bob's fear of HIV had diminished to a level of concern, caution, or perhaps what could be labeled a degree of anxiety. In fact, this fear reduction may have been beneficial for Bob, as a high level of fear is ineffectual in changing and maintaining health behaviors, and his prior mental connection of sex with death would be somewhat detrimental if maintained over time. Moreover, fear reduction can serve as a positive reinforcer for a behavior such as using condoms (Hovland, Janis, and Kelley 1953; Leventhal, Meyer, and Gutmann 1980; Sutton 1982). But contrary to educational phrases such as "fear is our worst enemy," a low level of fear or anxiety may be advantageous and adaptive to a dangerous environment in which a virulent virus lies in wait to transmit itself (Leventhal, Meyer, and Gutmann 1980; Levinton 1989). Put simply, when it comes to sex and HIV infection, the query is not should a gay man have fear or no fear; the real question is fuzzier—that is, how much fear or anxiety is optimal for him to maintain risk-reduction behaviors?

I met this guy [John]. It's funny because I saw him one day at the North Sidney swimming pool. I felt like, "Oh, this is it." When I first saw him at the pool, I didn't even try to say hello to him. A few weeks later I saw him again, this time at a gay bar. It was total physical attraction, but he left before I could say hello. Finally I saw him another time at the same bar about a month later and introduced myself. He was a very sweet guy. American, it turned out. He had been married for ten years, got divorced, and moved overseas. We started seeing each other and spent a lot of romantic weekends together.

We always used condoms, except of course for sucking. I guess I may have wanted to have unsafe sex, but I was too afraid. Not like I was before though—you know, freaked out. Maybe it was more like being cautious. As time passed on, the less fearful I think I became and the safer I felt.

Like I told you, it was total physical attraction with him. He had a great body and he was great in bed. You know, it was like his hands were always in the right place, whether on my legs, back, thighs, or dick. It wasn't clumsy sex like when you have to grab his hand and tell him what to do. He just knew. It was all just good, safe sex. Condoms [for anal sex] and sucking, but never boring.

Within six months of Bob's return to West Hollywood, John followed. During that six-month interval, Bob abstained completely from sex, but he was tempted several times. He was devoted, at least sexually, to John, but in spite of his fidelity, the intense affinity waned not too long after John landed, and Bob ended the relationship.

Afterward, Bob moved in and out of transient relationships. Although he persisted in his condom use for occasional anal sex, he preferred to substitute anal sex with oral sex as he considered oral sex to be safer. He also commenced using "heavy" drugs and began to drink "a lot" of alcohol. But despite this, he was capable of consistently practicing safer sex (see Bolton 1992; Weatherburn et al. 1993).

I moved back to West Hollywood and six months later John moved too. During that six months I was so much in love I just couldn't bring myself to have sex. Which for me was like . . . I still can't believe it. And this one boy—cute, cute, cute!—wanted me so bad. I just couldn't believe I didn't have sex with him, but that was the way it was.

When John moved to the States, I quit my job, and this is when I started using heavy drugs. I was unemployed for a long time. John got a job in San Francisco, and so we moved up there. I started doing ecstasy and party drugs. I smoked pot on a daily basis, and I started partying a lot. I guess I was trying to hide the pain of all those deaths or maybe I was unhappy with John. I don't know. We still practiced safer sex though, and I was only having sex within the relationship at this point. I did finally get a job that lasted about nine months and then quit again. My drug addiction got worse, and toward the end of the relationship, I started sleeping around, but most of my sleeping around was beating off and sucking, especially with people I didn't know, so it was pretty much safe. John wanted to settle down and move to the suburbs, but I couldn't deal with it. I left him and moved back to West Hollywood. This was in 1992.

Between 1992 and 1994, Bob's life changed, a change he claims to have been a breakthrough in his self-definition and his current social and financial success. After enlisting family support, he joined Alcoholics Anonymous (AA), became sober, and searched for a lover relationship. However, his desire for a relationship probably had little to do with his personal wants but instead was an attempt to emulate his older gay brother, and, in the end, Bob could not commit to one person.

After I moved back to West Hollywood, I slept around a lot, but practically gave up fucking. Just sucking. I did date a couple of guys for about six months or so, but they didn't work out. I have a really hard time with commitment. My brother's in a committed relationship. He's been in a relationship for four years. He and his lover bought a house together, but he has never fixed me up with anyone. But, yeah, he's like in a stable and monogamous relationship. His lover is just like one of the family, and comes to family get-togethers like Christmas and Thanksgiving. That would be nice for me to have something like what my brother has. Like I said, I have a hard time with commitment though. Although I'm probably a lot further along to a state where I can potentially make a commitment. . . . I think it has something to do with me being sober. . . .

Being sober is very important to me. Maybe it [getting sober] had something to do with my friend Bill, another friend who got sick about this time. I had to take care of him, and I spent a lot of time with Bill. Bill was a big drug addict, an alcoholic type, and always had lots of fun pharmaceuticals. We'd just get fucked up, and I'd like hook up his IV's. So I was doing some good work, you know, and I realized that I was destroying my life at the same time. I told myself "OK, after Bill dies get your shit together." It took him forever to die. He was around 120 pounds and then dropped down to 70 pounds. It was just unbelievable. After he died, I couldn't stop doing drugs. It got worse and worse—

really bad. So finally, a little over a year ago, my sister came down to help me, sort of held my hand and got me to an [AA] meeting. I've been sober since then. So you know, in my first year of sobriety I hadn't really . . . you know, it's funny . . . You're not supposed to get into a relationship [in AA] because you're supposed to get sober and that's all. Well, my brother was talking to me a couple of weeks ago, and he asked me, "So are you dating anybody?" I told him, "No, I'm not really dating anybody," but it's the most interesting thing. On the one hand, I feel like I'm farther away from a relationship than I have ever been because there is nobody that I'm interested in, but on the other hand, I feel like I'm closer to a relationship than I've ever been because I'm closer to myself than I've ever been. Because I don't need it, I feel like something will come along.

Sex, Relationships, and AIDS: Today and Tomorrow

I asked Bob to describe what a lover relationship—that "something" that "will come along"—means to him. In describing the perfect relationship, he veered away from his earlier stated desires to emulate his brother. Unlike his brother's situation, in Bob's fantasy relationship emotional commitment, sexual monogamy, and calcified stability are glaringly absent. Instead he emphasizes independence and change, and his ideal relationship would allow him to maintain his new sense of self.

One of the things I'm really looking for is growth and change. One of the things about a relationship I don't like is for it to be static. I have learned some things about love and commitment, but I like change. I like growth. There's so many people these days that . . . well you leave Los Angeles and come back a few years later, and all these people are exactly the same. They're doing the same thing. They're not any different. So I'm really looking for someone who is going to add something to my life because I feel like I've got a lot to offer. A lot of talents. A lot of interests. A way of looking at the world.

I do want somebody to share these with, but I don't want it to be a one-way street. I don't want to have somebody who I'm dominant over. I want somebody who's really independent and who has his own group of friends but shares my friends. Some people are in relationships and they've got separate groups of friends. Or some people think. "If we're together then all our friends are the same and your friends are my friends." That kind of mentality. I don't want it like that. I want us to have a separate life, but some of the same shared goals. I don't care if they have money or not. I've got enough money for myself. I'm certainly not looking for someone to take care of me or for someone who wants me to take care of them.

Bob did not mention a desired physical type, but I asked him later on, "What is your physical ideal for a lover or a sex partner?"

> I've been told that I don't have a type and that my taste in men is fast. I like some white boys. I like some Latin boys, you know. I'd really like someone from another country, but you never know, I might end up with some Waspy boy. By boy, I don't mean young, necessarily. It's just a phrase I use instead of man. It's sort of common. I do prefer my own age, maybe a little bit younger, but not too young. I like darker complexions, a good athletic physical shape—not fat or skinny—and white teeth. Sort of preppie, but not effeminate. Penis size doesn't matter so much with me. Really my type varies though. I mean there really isn't an overly specific type.

Bob recently had sex with someone he describes as the "perfect physical" man. He was Hispanic, early thirties, about Bob's height (5'4"), and "tight with muscles, a European build." The sex was oral only (both giving and receiving). Even though he does not like condoms for oral sex, he does take other precautions to reduce his risk of infection, and oral sex without a condom continues to be a risk-reduction strategy for him. Since not using a condom is both more physically and emotionally gratifying, he usually chooses to have oral sex "skin to skin" instead of having anal sex with a condom (see Davies et al. 1993). Just like when he was fooling around with other cub scouts as a young boy, mutual masturbation is not "real sex" and thus not a favored option. Real sex is penetration. Nonetheless, on those rare occasions when Bob feels the urge to have unprotected anal sex, his "internal voice" prevents him from completing the act.

> I don't use condoms when I give head or suck a boy off. I don't take cum in my mouth if I can prevent it, but sometimes it happens when I'm excited, the sex is fast, and the guy is holding my head. I do think it [HIV] is hard to get [orally] even if you swallow cum. I try not to fuck or get fucked.
>
> Mostly, like I said, I try to just give and get head. I don't really feel

that puts me at risk. I've gotten to the point that it's [anal penetration] just not worth it to me. As great as the sex might be, it's just not worth it. That's what I tell myself—or my little voice in my head tells me—when someone starts to fuck me without a condom or I start to fuck someone. It's not worth it, and I make them [the sex partner] stop and ask them to use a condom. Sometimes when I let someone fuck me, they might start and barely get in, but then I stop them and say, "you know, do you want to put on a condom?" And they always do.

Sometimes they get a little embarrassed or say "it doesn't feel as good." And I go "that's too bad." That doesn't hold water with me. It may be true, but it just isn't worth it. But this only happens if we've been going at it for a while: petting, heavy kissing, sucking, and the like. I don't talk about condoms before sex, but if I see it coming, I make them stop and put one on. Other times I'll suggest that we just do oral sex, especially if there are no condoms available. Sucking still lets me make that connection with skin. Even if I don't see the person again very often or never see them again, I feel like I've made some kind of, you know, connection. Sucking gives me a rush. I tried it with a condom once and I just don't get that rush. There's no connection when it's lip to rubber. . . .

Swallowing cum doesn't necessarily make the connection any better though. It's skin to skin. That's the connection. I've never had anyone ask me to wear a condom when I get head. They just don't. I don't think anyone does. Condoms for fucking, now, that's different. Well, Joe used to fuck me all the time [early to mid-1980s]. You remember, my friend who died. Another guy who died also used to fuck me. They were both sick and I was having sex with them. I couldn't believe that I wasn't infected. But by some divine power, I'm still negative. I've been very lucky.

Bob told me that he no longer associates sex with death, and he does not think about his friends who have died, people with AIDS, or "anything morbid" during sex. He enjoys sex now, and unlike the other men in this book, he seems to have a personalized cognitive method (the little voice) for controlling his behavior.

Experiences with Death and People Living with AIDS

Bob possesses a long history with AIDS. He feels this history, though tragic, has positively altered his life . He may feel somewhat

guilty or "ashamed" for being HIV negative, but his guilt is a moti-
vator to participate in volunteer work, not a drive to get infected
(see Odets 1995).

> Since AIDS, I've learned a lot about medicine. You know, I can talk to
> a doctor and really know what I'm talking about. I've learned a lot
> about love, and I take nothing for granted. I think I've learned a lot
> about myself in terms of my ability to deal with some very difficult
> issues. You know, somebody asked me, "Why do you volunteer with
> all yours friends sick?" I said, "It's for me." I was so frustrated early
> on, feeling like there was nothing I could do about it. I finally decided
> that I have to help. I felt guilty because I ran away from it when Joe
> was sick. I really felt bad about it. I felt some shame around it. I do it
> [volunteer] for myself because it gets me out of my head and I appre-
> ciate what I've got. It keeps me alive. I've gotten an extraordinary
> amount out of AIDS, and I've met some of the most wonderful people
> working with AIDS. Volunteering has given me some . . . well, it has
> made me face it. When I think of some of the best times I've spent, I
> think about people with AIDS.
>
> On the one hand, it's frustrating because I'm investing an incredi-
> ble amount of emotional energy on somebody who won't be here
> soon. On the other hand, people who don't have a lot of time left don't
> waste time. Like, for example, my friend Ronnie. I had been out of
> town and I got back on a Sunday. A friend called and told me that
> Ronnie was really very sick and in the hospital. I was leaving town
> again the next day, and so I went to see him. There were four other
> people visiting him. . . . So we were all visiting, "blah, blah, blah, blah."
> Then one guy left and then another, and pretty soon it was just me and
> Ronnie. I got up in the bed, sat down, and held his hand. We talked
> about two or three hours and just had the best quality time. Really got
> down to the heart of things. You know, you live in a place like West
> Hollywood where there's so much fluff and surface that it's kind of
> rare when you can communicate with someone on a really high level.
> He helped me so much that afternoon, just listening to him.
>
> I'm a big believer that you do a lot of your grieving while your
> friend is still here. I find that spending time with a friend while they
> are sick makes it much easier at the end. Just this morning, I was walk-
> ing down the street under the palm trees and I saw a friend that I
> haven't seen in a while. From looking at him—he looked pretty bad—
> I knew that it was time to start grieving again.

Amidst his grieving, Bob pursues his life as do many HIV-negative gay men. He works, loves, laughs, and provides comfort to others. And if his "little voice in his head" persists, his behavior change to safer sex may very well allow him to relish these human endeavors for the remainder of this century and into the next.

4 Phil: Binge and Purge

Do not defile yourselves in any of these ways, for these are the things that the heathen do.

—Leviticus 18:24

Sex is fun [for Bonobo chimpanzees, humankind's closest relatives]. Sex makes them feel good

—Meredith Small, "What's Love Got to Do with It?" (1992)

Despite his muscular two hundred pounds and 6′1″ height, thirty-eight-year-old Phil is frightened, afraid of becoming infected with HIV. With hopes of having his fears abated, Phil attended an HIV prevention workshop at a local AIDS organization where he picked up one of my flyers and arranged for an interview. I met with Phil on two different occasions at his condominium. He masked his fear well at our first meeting. He appeared calm, displaying no nervous twitches or mannerisms, and his softly inflected midwestern voice betrayed no hint of dread as it streamed from beneath an impressive raven-colored handlebar mustache.

Phil's condominium was crammed with fake objets d'art and imitation art deco furniture. A tall rose-colored vase sat poised on the entryway's gleaming hardwood floors, and track lighting ushered visitors into the main quarters. Numerous pictures of family members and of small groups of men—one with Phil raising a cocktail glass and laughing into the camera—rested here and there in the living room. Seemingly out of place in this elaborate decor, a wooden cross hovered over a stucco fireplace.

In a surrealistic flash, a big-screened television and a mahogany-stained entertainment center—the main focus of the living room—quickly distracted me from the antique cross. I noticed Phil's lineup of videos, stacked like books, some bearing obvious pornographic titles. With apparent care, the pornographic films were neatly arranged between a variety of other nonpornographic videos. I recognized a few of the video titles as vintage, gay pornography from the 1970s and early 1980s: "Kansas City Trucking Company" and "El Paso Wrecking Company," to name a couple. Other titles contained words such as "hard," "buns," "sex," and the like. Phil clearly, as was confirmed in the interview, took pleasure from pornography.

During the interview we sat across from each other at the narrowest portion of his oblong glass-topped dining room table. We were separated only by my small tape recorder. He eyed the device cautiously at first, but soon seemed to forget its humming existence as he became quite animated. Once he even gave a startled jump when the recorder clicked, a signal for me to turn the tape over.

Childhood

Phil was born in Chicago in 1956 to a traditional Italian Catholic family. The last of five children, and the only boy, he described his childhood in one word: discipline. In his parents' household, children were obedient. Gender roles were rigid if not downright oppressive. Any deviation from traditional expectations was not tolerated by his father or his mother, and in fact his mother was the primary disciplinarian. Phil's relationship with his mother, though not an affectionate one, was, in spite of her authoritarian role, more substantial than his relationship with his father (see Herdt 1989).

> Mother was the homemaker. She'd thought about going to work in an office once, but my aunts told her that her place was at home with her children. She always did what my aunts said to do. They were my father's sisters and watched my mother's every move. My father wore the pants in the family, and my aunts enforced his rules. Mother didn't wear the pants in the family, but she did control the discipline of the children. Slapping and spanking were normal back then. I guess it'd be called child abuse nowadays, but I think we were properly reared. We were taught respect, to be polite to people, and to be considerate of

others. We were taught to be honest and not to lie—except at the market, just a little, if it'd get us a good deal. I did lie to my mother sometimes. I had to, especially about sexuality and about anything else she might consider sinful.

With my sisters' help, mother did all the cooking and cleaning. Mother was proud of her house, but my aunts would come over and inspect her work, and if one thing was not perfect—absolutely perfect—they'd make a comment, going on and on about how hard my father, the lawyer, worked.

Father came home from work and we ate supper at seven every night. Always at seven. He was a traditional Italian man, and there was no physical affection doled out. My father was always working or hanging out with my uncles and his men friends, so he didn't spend much time with me. Don't get me wrong. He was proud to have a boy to carry on the family name, but . . . come to think of it, I don't think I ever even hugged my mother until she was over sixty years old. I know this sounds horrible, but it really wasn't so bad. I knew they both loved me because . . . I don't know . . . I just knew, but I was closer to my mother than to my father. Mother had more time for me.

As far as my sisters, well, they were girls and we led separate lives as was tradition.

Phil was well liked by his peers. Even though he was "slightly effeminate" in mannerisms and speech, he did not suffer abuse from other children; but as a "sissy," he discerned that he was somehow unlike other boys. However, as is typical of gender-nonconforming boys, he had no idea what to call this difference (see Green 1985, 1987). The apparent lack of peer harassment for behavioral differences could be related to the constraints of Phil's peer group membership as his childhood acquaintances were restricted by religion and parental affiliations.

I played with girls a lot. My dad used to tell people that girls were all over me, but I just liked the games they were playing. I was never good at sports, but I always took girls to dances and we learned how to ballroom dance. I had music lessons and that kind of thing. I had a very nice circle of friends and we did a lot together. My parents would get together with their parents while we rode bikes, went to the movies, or what have you. We were a close-knit little Italian Catholic group, and we all went to the same Catholic schools from elementary to high school.

As Phil grew older and discovered adolescent sex, his sexual partners, both male and female, came from this "close-knit little Italian Catholic group."

> We played childhood games. I guess you'd call them sexual. Mainly I played with girls, displaying my penis and chasing them. They'd giggle and sometimes let me touch their panties. We were exploring. With little boys I didn't get a lot of experience because most of my friends were girls. Except when I was eight one of the neighbor boys wanted me to masturbate him. I sort of stared at his penis and told him that I thought it was a sin. He zipped up, and I swore never to tell anyone, because if I did, he would beat me up. When we all grew older and got into our teens, I dated some of the girls, and by then I was also having sex with boys. Everybody was having sex with everybody. We were quite the young heathens. If I was having sex with a guy, I was probably having sex with his sister too.

Before reaching his teens, Phil was "molested" at the age of twelve by a man who he believes was in his forties, but he is not certain. Phil did not and does not perceive this episode to have been abusive. For him, it was an exhilarating experience, and he harbors no apparent regrets for its occurrence.

> It was 1968. I'll never forget it. It was really hot and humid. Chicago summers can be a carnival of misery. Anyway, I went to see a movie, some "B" movie, playing at a theater. I was sitting toward the back of the theater and this man sat down beside me. There were plenty of empty seats in the place and I thought him sitting there, right up next to me, to be a little odd, but I was only twelve; and kids don't think about danger. So I sat for a little bit, but then I started to get up and move. I just wanted some privacy and I guess I maybe felt a little awkward sitting there. The man put his hand on my leg and asked me where I was going. I was polite and said, "to the bathroom." He told me to wait a second and grabbed my hand. He put my palm on his lap, and he had an erection. It wasn't too big, as I recall, but just sort of small really: maybe six inches, tops. I freaked and ran as fast as I could. My heart was pounding really hard, but not in a bad way. I was just excited. I ran to my room, and believe it or not I had a hard-on. So I masturbated a couple of times or so while thinking about [that experience].
>
> The next day, I went back to the theater and he was there again. I sat two seats away. He started masturbating, and I moved over and finished it for him. He took my penis out too and played with it, but

I didn't come. I guess I was afraid of getting caught. When I got home and saw my mother, I felt so guilty—being Catholic, don't you know. Then I felt sort of sick because I wondered if she ever did that to [masturbated] my dad. I became curious, but I never went back to that theater. I was scared to go back. I don't know why. I was just scared to go back.

I don't think what happened was sexual abuse at all, but I guess some people would probably think so. After all, I encouraged him the second time, and I'm really glad it happened. Whoever he is—I've nicknamed him Mr. Thimble because of his dick size—I am grateful. It was like my initiation. I became a man, well . . . sort of one. But I still thought God was going to punish me, especially when my mother's eyes used to look at me real stern-like, as if she knew. It was a mix of guilt and happiness.

Coming Out

In contrast to experiencing coming out as a continuous process (Herdt 1992), Phil remembers having had many separate and sporadic coming out events (Henrickson 1994). For Phil, each time he declares his gay identity, he views it as coming out all over again (Cain 1991).

The first time I came out was when I wanted to become a priest. Oh yes, I wanted to be a priest. Can you believe it—me, the little boy who masturbated a dirty old man in a theater? When I decided to be a priest, I was about nineteen years old and kind of stupid. So I went to see a priest, partly to discuss it with him and then to discuss this desire I had to have sex with other men. I didn't think I could be a priest until I did something about this desire, and I thought the priest would help me to change. But instead he wanted to have sex. And we did. By sex I mean oral stuff, because I didn't know there was any other way to have sex with a man at that time. After that, I figured that the priesthood couldn't cure me. I was a kid. I wasn't really stupid.

To make a long story short, I did not become a priest. I decided I'd try to get married instead. Come to think of it, I was really attracted to all the protocol of weddings—gifts, the whole thing including a lot of hoopla. I wanted to have a big wedding, and I did in 1976; but the marriage only lasted a year. My ex-wife Margaret—she's still my friend and we chat on the phone sometimes—when I told her I was gay, that was the second time I came out. I told her that I was gay and we should try to get our marriage annulled. I didn't have sex with a man the whole time we were married, but I sure wanted to. I thought if marriage couldn't change my attraction to men, then nothing could. So I came out to her, and for the first time in my life I moved into my own place. Then I came out several more times that year. I started telling anyone and everyone. I'm surprised I didn't announce it from the rooftops.

Sex and Relationships Before AIDS

After his divorce in 1978, Phil worked for a Chicago department store creating window displays, an occupation that allowed him to make connections with other gay men in the retail industry. Possibly induced by his childhood theater experience, in Chicago he started frequenting a gay movie theater to seek out sex with other men.

> I was itching to have sex. I discovered a movie theater where people were having sex in the dark. I went twice a week and would suck guys off or get sucked off. I never had anything but oral sex with a man until I was twenty-three years old because of the places I went for sex—movie theaters and such places. You can give and get a blow job standing up or sitting down. You can do it with your clothes on, and it's easy to clean up afterwards. So oral sex it was.

Phil began to fraternize with other gay employees at the department store where he worked, and by 1979 he had stopped patronizing pornographic movie theaters. At this point, he immersed himself in a gay clique and acquired a "discerning taste" for older men and anal sex.

> I started meeting men who were older than me—not too old, just in their thirties and forties. Some of them had money and they all knew each other. They ran in the same circles more or less. I got hooked up with this group by way of some of the gay guys and a girl from work. I guess you'd call her [the girl from work] a fag hag because all her friends were gay men. We just called her "girlfriend." . . .
> The older men treated me nicely. They took me to restaurants and spent money on me. I became a bottom [anal receptive] because I was always the younger one. I wish I could say that was still the case these days. Occasionally one of them [the older men] would throw their

legs up, but that was a treat for me. I like it both ways really. I'm very versatile, as they say. . . . Safer sex? Oh well, we didn't know about AIDS then. We just fucked and fucked. Who cared? Drugs flowed, and I dropped acid for the first time, sniffed poppers, smoked pot, and all that. I was trying all kinds of new things just like a kid in school. I felt grown up and was experiencing—I don't know what—a renaissance I guess.

In 1980 I fell in love with an attorney—just like my father, don't you know—who was part of the group that I ran with. We moved in together and had a monogamous relationship. I quit my job, stayed home, took care of the house, and did other wifely duties—had his martini ready when he got home and pasta on the stove. I didn't cheat on him. I was dedicated to Jeff just like my mother had always been to my father. Thank God, he didn't have sisters to inspect everything. My poor mother. My aunts really kept her on her toes when I was growing up. . . . Anyway, in 1982 Jeff and I moved to Los Angeles.

Sex and Relationships After AIDS

Phil and his lover Jeff relocated to Los Angeles after Jeff accepted a new job as a tax attorney. They bought a house in the Silver Lake area of Los Angeles. Silver Lake, an area described by E. Michael Gorman (1992) as "West Hollywood's cross-town rival for cultural hegemony in Los Angeles's gay male world," sits to the east of West Hollywood. It is an older residential area of Los Angeles, and the gay men who live there tend to be more "couple-oriented" and somewhat older than their West Hollywood counterparts.

This move marked a dramatic turn in Phil's life as at least two important events interrupted his rhythmic, "monotonous" day-to-day existence. It was after the relocation to Silver Lake that Phil had his first encounter with AIDS, and the dynamics of his relationship with Jeff took a downturn.

We found a cute little house overlooking the reserve [a lakelike water reserve in Silver Lake]. The house was beautiful, and I immediately decorated it to suit my taste. I made friends with some of the neighbors, but unlike in Chicago, I couldn't get a morning coffee clutch going. LA queens are much more in their own little world, if you know what I mean. Then, I think it was in 1983 that one of my neighbors came down with pneumonia. We all thought it was just pneumonia, but it got worse and worse. He really caught himself a fever and couldn't even get out of bed. It scared the living hell out of me. As you can probably guess, it was something much, much more than pneumonia. It was AIDS. That was my first time seeing somebody like that. We were all scared. It was AIDS and people freaked out. Some gay couples even stopped having dinner parties because they were afraid the disease would get on their fine china and hop off onto them. It wasn't that they were bad people. It was just that everybody was scared shitless back then.

My relationship with Jeff was strained, but not because of AIDS. We were just losing interest in each other. We were in a same-old-thing, everyday slump, and we stopped having sex, so I wasn't getting any [sex]. I didn't mind at first, but later it began to drive me nuts. I bought porno magazines and kept them stashed away. I'd masturbate in the bathroom just to get a release. I couldn't stand not having sexual relations for very long.

I moved out, got a small, little bachelor pad above a garage in West Hollywood, and Jeff eventually sold the house. My lifestyle was cut way back. I worked two retail jobs for a while and eventually made manager, as I am today.

After he and Jeff separated in 1984, Phil, coming off a year of "not having sex with anything but my right hand," partook of numerous evenings filled with sexual pleasure, continuing a life pattern of long periods of abstention from sex with other men (purging) followed by short episodes of binge sex. Earlier in his life, abstention appears to have been a response to gender expectations and religious guilt, but now his fear of AIDS supplanted, or at least accentuated, these earlier sexual constraints.

Uhm, uhm ... Now you're probably going to think I was a total slut or something, but I went totally wild. I worked a lot, but I partied hard during the week and weekend nights. Work and party, that was all I did. I took up easy drugs again like pot and sometimes cocaine when I could afford it. I wasn't an abuser at all. I couldn't have afforded to be one if I'd wanted to. I just liked a toke or a snort now and then when I was in a party mood.

AIDS was around and I was still sort of scared, but I wasn't using condoms yet. You know what was *bee*-zarre? I started dating men my own age or especially younger. My taste in men wasn't so strict, after all. So I was the top most of the time now. I'd fuck them. Maybe that's why I didn't get infected. Not that I didn't get poked from time to time, but it just seemed that young guys wanted me to do it because . . . well, you don't want to hear this, do you? Or Do you? [*I nod*] My penis is very large and they seemed to like that.

Then I had sex with this guy, I think it was 1985 but I'm not sure. He turned out to have AIDS. I wigged out, don't you know, and didn't touch anyone for a very, very long time. That's when I really started building up my porno collection.

Phil went through quite a few cycles of pleasure-seeking followed by abstinence brought on by fears of infection, but the episodes of actual sexual encounters became increasingly infrequent over time and ever shorter in duration. This culminated into his current sexual pattern: drawn-out periods of masturbation at home with his extensive collection of pornography interspersed with occasional sexual encounters.

I started staying home and stopped doing just about anything socially, except with friends from work or with a couple of close girlfriends in my building. Over the last few years I've bought all those porno flicks that I showed you. I like them. I like them because the next morning I don't have to worry about getting tested [for HIV] and I don't feel guilty. Not at all. I just wish they could satisfy me. My life would be so much, well, simpler don't you think. . . . I don't know, but sometimes I want to touch somebody else's dick, not just mine. You know, make some kind of human sexual contact and not just use my hand. I just have to do it. And when I go out to get it—with all those stored-up hormones a-hoppin'—I just go wild.

Sex and Relationships: Today and Tomorrow

Besides his binge-and-purge sexual pattern, Phil also discussed his views on long-term relationships. Phil does not want another lover relationship because he feels that it would stifle his emotional growth.

Since Jeff, I've grown up a lot. I can't believe I played the housewife role. I guess that's what I thought gay men like me were supposed to do. Today I just do my own thing. I have my condo, and I have a good job managing the [department] store. I really don't need another person, and I don't want to play in a lover role. I want to be myself, not part of another person. . . . I mean . . . I am just now finding my independence again. Once I feel like I have found myself, maybe I'll settle down again. But if that ever happened—and I doubt it will—it would be very different from my previous relationship. I won't be the husband or the wife. Sometimes I think it would be great to have a steady sex partner. But the emotional commitment, I'm not ready for that. No. I don't think I'm ready for that again. Not right now anyway. Maybe later on in the future.

Although he is not looking for a relationship, Phil does have an ideal physical type for potential sexual partners, or "fuck buddies." His description of an ideal physical type closely resembles the contemporary look of gay pornographic and erotica actors and models. While describing this fantasy partner to me, Phil went over to his video collection, pulled one from the shelf, and proudly showed me a video cover's photograph of a porn star who resembled his verbal description.

If I had a fuck buddy, I would like him to be about twenty-nine or thirty, maybe as old as thirty-five, just a little younger than me. Like I said, after I left Jeff I sort of took on younger men, but not chicken [very young gay men]. He would have blond hair, kind of a short cut. He'd be stocky and muscular, not fat. I don't like body hair like I used to. I like them smooth. So he'd be shaven except for his pubic hair. I'm not into shaving men. He'd do it to himself. I'm not that kinky. . . . And penis size, oh I'd say average to large. I don't find small penises to be very sexy. I know that sounds awfully tacky, but I just don't.

Despite his extensive selection of celluloid fantasies available at the push of a button, Phil seeks out his fantasy man during his bingeing evenings. And regardless of the degree of risk taken during a binge, he "always" feels guilty afterward. Driven by this guilt, he once attended Sexual Compulsives Anonymous, a group that believes sex to be an addiction and that is modeled on the twelve-step Alcoholics Anonymous program.

I feel like I am out of control. It's like I'm so hypersexual. I guess it might be an addiction. I attended Sexual Compulsives Anonymous a few times, but it didn't seem to help. I guess I wanted a quick fix, but I'm not sure it's an addiction anyway. Maybe my Catholic background makes me feel guilty about sex, but now there's a virus out there, a deadly virus, and it scares the hell out of me. Sex feels good when I'm doing it, but I'm so scared sometimes: the next day . . . when I wake up.

Phil's fear of HIV is so powerful that he appears to be trapped in an all-or-nothing sexual straitjacket. Over the past two years, he has "binged" (a binge being one encounter) at least five times. On three of these occasions he had anal sex as the penetrator and did not use a condom. He characterizes these binge sex events as being "wild and out of control."

For Phil, an all-or-nothing approach (sex/no sex) appears not to be, and certainly has not been, advantageous. Indeed, such an approach is likely to reinforce his binge/purge pattern by not allowing some type of safer release of his "hypersexuality." Learning to cope with his fear and to manage or moderate his sexual encounters may lead to a better solution (Hovland, Janis, and Kelley 1953; Leventhal, Meyer, and Gutmann 1980; Sutton 1982). I will expand on this approach in the final chapter.

In spite of his self-described "hypersexuality," on two of his five binge escapades Phil managed to use a condom for anal sex. I asked him to compare and contrast his most recent noncondom experience (less than a month before the interviews) with his most recent condom experience (seven months before the interviews). His experience without the condom proved more vivid in his mind than his experience with a condom, probably owing to the differing lengths of time that have elapsed since these events.

In any case, his experience of penetration without a condom contrasted markedly with his experience with one. He seemed to relish the former more so than he did the latter. When relating his noncondom experience, he grinned, displaying bleached-white teeth, and his face became flushed.

Due to his larger-than-average penis, condoms are somewhat uncomfortable and tight for Phil, and thus he quite naturally finds greater pleasure in his experience without wearing one. Further, for his last unsafer encounter, the description of his partner is reminiscent of that of his fantasy partner, and the entire experience was characterized by the acting out of a pornographic film scene. Foreplay went on for a longer time, and both he and his partner were more aggressive.

Although condoms were available in both the safer and unsafer instances, Phil's partner put the condom on Phil in the safer encounter, while in the unsafer encounter Phil's inebriated partner en-

couraged him to continue without one after Phil had already penetrated. Phil complied with this latter partner's pleas and did not
stop, but even though highly aroused, he still succeeded in pulling
out before ejaculation.

Despite their differences, the two events share some similarities.
For example, Phil met both partners at a bar—although they were
different bars—and he did not discuss safer sex with either of them
or inquire about their HIV status before getting on with the sexual acts.

The Safer Episode

I met him [the partner in which a condom was used] at a bar. I wasn't
drunk or nothing like that. He was cute enough I suppose. I remember
he had a nice round butt and may have been in his thirties. It was
really quick. We went to his place and I was in and out, so to speak.
There was a lot of oral sex at first, but mainly he sucked me. Like I said,
my penis is pretty large, ten inches more or less, and it's thicker than
the average. So they [sexual partners] usually like to do me, especially
if they're a size queen [a gay man who prefers large penises].

This man wasn't really great. Nothing to write home about. He
was blond, tall, and a little hairy but not too much. While I was on
his bed and he was doing me, he stopped and put a condom on me.
It's difficult because condoms are always tight on me and they sometimes hurt a little. But he was successful and climbed on and rode. I
rolled him over and kept going. There wasn't a whole lot to it. I've
seen him around since. He says "hi" when we bump into each other,
but I don't think we'll do it again. I'm always afraid that I'll want
more sex.

The Unsafer Episode

A few weeks ago, I picked up this young guy, late twenties, at the Rage
[a West Hollywood gay bar]. He was so hot, and as usual I was really
horny. He had blond hair and a perfectly shaven muscular physique.
He was just a little shorter than me, maybe up to my nose. I didn't have
to stoop to kiss him. We had a couple of drinks and came back here to
my place. He was a little drunk. I guess he'd been at the bar for a while.
While I was getting him something more to drink in the kitchen, he
saw my porno collection, so I put one [a video] on to get us worked up
a little.

He was great. He wanted to do one of the porno fantasies. I mean like act one out. I thought it was a little weird but I went along with it. In the film we were watching, this young guy was caught beating off in a bathroom by a janitor. This little man [Phil's sexual partner] even wanted to know if I had some coveralls to put on so I'd look more like a janitor, but I didn't. He went into the bathroom with one of my porno magazines and masturbated. I peeked in the door and watched for—I don't know for sure—maybe ten . . . fifteen minutes. Then I walked in and deepened my voice: "Hey, what are you doing?" He looked surprised and asked me if I wanted to help. . . . We played in the bathroom for a while with a lot of talking like in porno movies. . . . I guess you'd call it talking trash. Then we went to the bedroom, and he got a little wild and wanted me to bite him. It was really kinky for me, but I was excited. I don't remember why, but I was so worked up that I just slipped in. And then he begged me to continue and I forgot . . . let me correct that . . . I didn't even think about a condom. I don't think I had one around, but he had one. I saw it when he emptied his pockets and took off his pants. I knew the sex felt better somehow, but I didn't want to stop and he kept me going, asking me to fuck him. . . . I pulled out before cumming though.

He stayed overnight, and the next day I asked him his HIV status. He said he was negative, but well, you know how that is. I hope he was telling the truth. We didn't talk about condoms at all. I just asked him if he was HIV negative or HIV positive. He called me later that day, but I let my phone machine answer. I felt so ashamed and guilty. I felt like I would probably feel if I'd gotten caught masturbating in a church or something. I really want to get this under control. I keep promising myself that it will never, ever happen again. I haven't had sex with another person since. . . . I went and got tested [for HIV] a couple of days later.

Phil knows that if he were infected, antibodies may not be detected on an HIV test until a few weeks or even months following exposure, but he took the test anyway, as other gay men sometimes do, to comfort themselves (see Phillips and Coates 1995; Phillips et al. 1995).

I don't know why I get tested right away. I know if I'm infected it might not show up yet. I guess it gives me something to do. Something to do and try and make it better. It made me feel better and gave me back a little control, or I guess it made me think I had more control.

Experiences with Death and People Living with AIDS

Phil's contacts with people living with AIDS have been minimal compared to the other men interviewed. Beyond the neighbor with AIDS whom he met when he first moved to Los Angeles and the person with AIDS with whom he had sex in 1985, he says that he has "only" lost one friend. He emphasized "only" as if he had not carried his own share of burden.

> I lost a friend back in 1993. We were close, I guess. We'd do things together on a Sunday afternoon every now and then—go shopping, have a drink, or just go down to the beach. When he got really sick, he moved back to the Midwest to be with his family. I helped him pack and said goodbye, but no, I don't know that many people who have died or who have AIDS. Like I said, I don't have a whole lot of friends anyway. I'm sort of a loner. I mean, I see people around like at the gym and then suddenly they're not around anymore. I might pick-up *Frontiers* or *Edge* [both West Hollywood gay-oriented magazines] and I'll recognize so-and-so's face in the obituaries. It is really scary, AIDS is . . . really scary. . . . I'm glad I'm HIV negative. So glad.

Given his history of risk-taking, I asked Phil how he felt about being HIV negative and what does he feel has contributed to his HIV negative status. He does not feel guilty about being HIV negative, just guilty about putting himself at risk, but he is still Catholic and believes God may play a role in protecting him from infection.

> I am so grateful to be HIV negative. [*He knocks on the table, performing the American folk ritual of "knocking on wood"*] I hope that I never have to go through those horrors [of AIDS]. It's really sad—really, really sad—all these young beautiful men dying. I want to live to be ninety-nine years old. My God, AIDS frightens me. If I got infected, I don't know what I would do. I wouldn't be able to handle it. I feel so sorry for them. It must be awful at the end. Really just plain awful. I had rather die in a car accident. It's quick. I really would, no matter how awful that sounds.
>
> God has protected me. Oh yes, I'm still religious. I pray to God, and I do believe he plays a role in keeping me HIV negative. I know that probably means he plays a role in others being HIV positive and that's an awful thought. But it might be true. I don't know for sure. It's not like he's punishing people by making them HIV positive. That's just a

bunch of fundamentalist Christian mumbo-jumbo. It's just that some people he takes away for whatever reason. We'll probably never understand it all, really. . . . I just know for sure that if I could just give up sex altogether, I know I could stay HIV negative. I've just got to get it under control.

At the end of the second interview, as I left Phil's company and headed toward my car, I became lost in my own thoughts, remembering an old female friend of mine whose weight fluctuated mercilessly throughout most of her life. In retaliation to the condemnation of "heavy" by her bathroom scales, she would jump from one all-or-nothing diet to another. For a while, she would do just fine, but if she weakened and gave in to one piece of chocolate cake, a dish of ice cream, or a even a cookie, the diet would be over. Eventually, beaten down by sentiments of defeat, she gave up dieting altogether. That memory gave me pause, and I shuddered to think.

5

Alexander: Knowing Better

Now as I watch the progress of the plague, the friends surrounding me
fall sick, grow thin, and drop away. Bared, is my shape less vague—
Sharply exposed with a sculpted skin.

—Thom Gunn, "The Missing" (1989)

The meeting of two personalities is like the contact of two chemical
substances. If there is any reaction, both are transformed.

—Carl Jung, *Man and His Symbols* (1964)

Forty-three-year-old Alexander is a social service provider at a small
AIDS agency. Given his work experience, he naturally understands
the risks associated with unprotected anal sex. Alexander has witnessed more than his share of the casualties that can result from taking such a risk. Despite this, however, he had had anal sex without a
condom as the receptive partner less than a month before our meeting.

I did not interview Alexander in my home, nor in his, but instead
I let him choose a neutral location where he would feel most comfortable. Yielding to his wishes, I met him in a quaint windowless
room polished with soft lighting that created a moody, dark, and
calming ambiance. We slumped into soft, cushy pale-green chairs,
snuggling into them as he talked. I jotted sporadic notes as my recorder hummed beneath the white noise of the air conditioner.
Alexander's voice bore a quiet lilt, and although his skin pigment is
somewhat dark, from time to time his complexion blushed a pinkish
hue beneath his thick black hair.

After the interview, he seemed refreshed. He offered his gratitude
for being allowed to participate in the study and described our meet-

ing as "therapeutic." It was the first time he had confessed to anyone his sexual gamble, and he felt that he "should have known better" than to throw the dice.

Childhood

When he was six months old, Alexander was adopted by a French couple, and his adoptive mother did not keep his birth circumstances a secret from him. Alexander was deeply bonded with his adoptive mother, and she played a prominent role in his early emotional development.

Though also physically affectionate, his relationship with his adoptive father was not the same as with his mother. The father and son relationship was more emotionally distant and removed (see Herdt 1989). According to Alexander, this discrepancy between physical and emotional connection is inherent in French culture in which physical, but not emotional, displays of affection are common between family members regardless of gender.

> The woman and man who adopted me were French like me, and I found out that I was adopted at an early age. My mom would say that I was from the stomach, and I would ask her if I was from her stomach. She'd say, "No, from your mother's stomach. She put you up for adoption because she wanted you to have a good home."
>
> I was very close to my adoptive mother. I guess I was a mama's boy to some degree because she took me—and my sister too—everywhere. If it was a funeral, we went. If it was a trip, we went. She never left us at home, and she liked to do things with us, probably because she couldn't have children of her own.
>
> I identified strongly with her. I had dark hair and brown eyes as she did, but my sister favored my dad. My mother was also strong and wore the pants in the family. She was from a big city, and my dad was from a little hick town, so mother was considered the wanton woman by my father's family, except by his parents, my grandparents. They actually liked her. The rest of his family thought she was a slut or something. She had some real pizzazz. I guess that I identified so strongly with her, because I knew I was different, somehow.
>
> She understood me and questioned what went on in my life. She'd ask me, "How do you feel?" But with my dad it was com-

pletely different. He was very closemouthed, and never really expressed his feelings. He could talk to people and shoot the breeze, but he never really expressed his feelings. But because my father was French, he was very physically affectionate. All my relatives were affectionate, especially the men, kissing and embracing each other when they said goodbye.

I too was and am exceptionally affectionate. I used to bite my cousin's hand and she would ask, "Why are you doing that?" And I would answer, "Because I love you." My mother would call me *le chou,* which is French for somebody who likes to lick. I was always affectionate and kissy.

Although Alexander's sister is a couple of years his junior, his relationship with her while growing up was more akin to a peer relationship than to a sibling relationship. This could be because his family relocated several times during his childhood, making it difficult for Alexander to establish a peer group. When outside friendships were made, both Alexander and his sister shared them as they played with the same children, playing games that at times consisted of sexual play.

Growing up my sister and I were very close, and we usually had the same friends. Our family moved around a lot because of my dad's job as a lumberjack, and it was hard to keep making new friends. As far as the friends that I did make, they were usually our neighbors, but there weren't many of them because we always lived in rural areas.

Neighborhood kids would sometimes pick on me because my English skills were poor. French was my first language, not English. They used to call me French Fry. And I was short. They teased me about that too. Kids can be rotten, but I don't remember being teased because I was different or a sissy of any sort, and I did have friends here and there.

I remember this one family that had three boys and two girls. We all used to hang out together, and I had a couple of cousins who didn't live too far away who would hang out with us [Alexander and his sister] too. That's when my sister and I did some sexual experimentation stuff with this boy Roger and his sister Nadine. My sister and I used to go with them into the woods where there were these abandoned cars. In the cars we pretended to do what adults did without fully understanding what the hell we were doing. Nadine, Richard, my sister, and I would be like humping each other. I had no clue. Whatever it was, we knew it was naughty, but we were all doing it and not relating it to . . . you know. . . . Boys do it one way and girls do it another way.

I guess Richard was my first sexual experience since he taught me how to masturbate. He said, "I just found out how to do this [masturbate]." He was rubbing his penis like a campfire stick between his two hands. And for a long time that was my favorite way to masturbate. I remember kind of like having an orgasm without anything coming out, just some fluid. It was fun, but then we moved away and I don't remember how it ended.

Notwithstanding his same-sex experiments with Richard, Alexander developed "crushes" on girls and sexually experimented with them as well.

I remember some other cousins who were girls. They were older adolescents—about seven years older as I recall, and they had big breasts. They used to like for me to play with them. It was a form of sexual molestation I guess, but I liked it. I didn't know the difference. I mean, here's your babysitter playing sexually with you. We just thought, "Oh well, it's nasty." We were raised Catholic. . . . So the whole thing around sexuality as a kid was that way [nasty] regardless of who I was with. All sex acts were bad. . . . I liked girls at the time, I guess. I had a girlfriend once and had a crush on a female teacher and all that like other boys.

Alexander feels that his childhood abruptly ended when he was eleven years old and the woman who he admired the most, his adoptive mother, died from breast cancer. From that moment forward, Alexander's role in the family changed from that of son/brother to a modified parent/wife, and he took on an enormous amount of responsibility for his age.

After my mother died from breast cancer, I felt abandoned. She and I were so close. After she died, I took on the role of parent for my younger sister. I was also the wife and spouse for my dad, in a family sense, not in a sexual sense. I guess I became an adult at an early age.

My dad was a good provider, but as a lumberjack he had to work long hours, and he didn't know how to discipline children or to pay the bills. Before she died, my mother always did these things. I had to try and remember what I had been taught by mom. At the same time, my sister and I needed some structure, so I created that structure. I became the parent.

Coming Out

Alexander's coming out process was twofold: coming out as bisexual followed by coming out as a gay man. Bisexuality was an acceptable label under which he could test out his homosexual desires—which in retrospect he believes were always there—and reveal these desires to others (Green 1985, 1987; Herdt 1989).

Relative to other gay men, Alexander believes that he was tardy in coming out as a gay man. He did not come out until he was twenty-four, subsequent to an interval of having sex with both men and women. But once he found other gay men, he was on his way. While in college, he combed through heterosexual erotic publications, and ironically it was there that he found a group of other men who shared his sexual urges.

I didn't come out until I was in college and twenty-four years old. I was late, but I had always known that I desired men; I just never had a label. I'd heard the words *gay* and *homosexual*, but I didn't know what they meant. I remember one time looking up the word *homosexual* in the dictionary and the definition was "a person who loves himself." So I thought, "That's me. I masturbate."

I didn't have sex in high school really. In college I had sex with some women, but it wasn't very satisfying. They [women] were very aggressive, and I didn't know what I was doing.

While I was still in school, I went to work at a hospital where I gave people baths and rubs. I remember that I used to get a hard-on when I bathed the men. I'd be aware of my erection, but I still didn't know what it was about, until one time, when I was giving this older guy a back rub, he turned around and grabbed my crotch. I gently took his hand and put it down. He was very embarrassed, and so was I.

I started reading *Penthouse Forum* and other magazines and found stories about gay men and women. I finally understood what *gay* meant, and it meant more—much more—than masturbation.

Then when I was giving another guy a bath rub, it happened again, but this time the guy was really hot. I realized then that I liked that. Thereafter I made a point to look through letters from bisexual people in *Penthouse Forum*. In there I found a hotline number. I called the hotline, and they gave me the name of a rap group for gay/bisexual men in New Hampshire. So I called, and I went. The next thing I knew, I was involved with this group of gay and bisexual men who were very open about sexuality, kind of like a Gay 101. I had sex with some of them, but not all. I learned a lot in the group. I found out about golden showers [urinating on another person], fisting [putting a hand or fist up another person's anus] and all those things. I learned about them before having sex with a lot of guys.

After I joined the group and found out where I could go to meet other men—bars, parks, and such places—I started having more sex with guys. I still thought that I was bisexual. I thought I could still have sex with a woman even though I had no desire to do so. I could probably even have sex with a woman now, but my preference is to only have sex with men; and it's a strong preference.

Within a short period of time after joining this group, Alexander came out as bisexual to his sister. Her response was positive and accepting, a response that may have been an impetus to continue the coming out process leading on to a gay identity.

When I was in college, I saw my sister reading a book about a priest who was gay, so I took a deep breath and told her that I was bisexual— I didn't quite identify as gay yet. Her response was a great big relief for me. She said, "Listen, I didn't want to burst your bubble, but I really wasn't worried about it." She's been very supportive and over the years has gotten more comfortable with it. She goes dancing with my lesbian friends, and she and her husband have accepted my friends like family.

Despite the acceptance of his sexuality by his sister, he never came out to his father, though he did make attempts to do so. Alexander's lack of success in telling his father seems to be related to the dearth of feeling in his father's emotional expressiveness and his father's general discomfort in discussing all matters related to sex and sexuality.

I wanted to tell my father. One day I asked him, "Do you ever wonder what's going on with my sister and me? Aren't you interested in who we're dating?" He said, "No." From that I assumed that he wasn't interested or didn't want to hear it. He never talked about sex. When I was young, I'd sometimes find his girlie magazines in the shed, but he'd never talk about them. He'd just get embarrassed and that was it.

Because of all that, I figured that it wasn't worth telling him. I have taken a couple of guys home, and he treated them just as any other friend. We slept in the same bed, but there was nothing out of the ordinary about it. It was no big deal.

Sex and Relationships Before AIDS

In the 1970s, Alexander "blossomed." As with many of the other men in this book, his coming out initiated an expansion of sexual boundaries as he explored his recently uncloaked desires. Although he had a couple of short-lived relationships, his thoughts and desires were for pleasure and finding lots of it.

> During college, I got drafted. It was 1972, the very last draft. It was also the year that President Nixon dropped all deferments, including college deferments. I didn't want to participate in the military, and it is obviously not "me." After all, I am no marine. I could have gotten out of it by being gay, but I wasn't accepting a gay label at that point. There were guys in my dorm who were not gay but said they were [homosexual] in order to get out of the draft. Instead, I declared myself a conscientious objector and did community service in a hospital, the same hospital I was already working in. I just had to go and do my duty. That was when I told you about being felt up by the guys that I bathed and gave back rubs to.
>
> After that, I met one guy in a bar, Peter. We became boyfriends or, I guess, lovers. I say "boyfriends" because we never really lived together. I wanted to have our own place to live, but he was still living with his parents. I got bored with him anyway. That's when I moved to Boston.
>
> I really blossomed in Boston. It was the late seventies. At that time, I was small and dark-haired and a lot of men found me attractive, so I never had to want for sexual partners. And I was very outgoing, sexually. I was ultra-flirtatious. I had a lot of sex. Literally lots of it. Those were the days when the more sex you had, the more popular you were. I used to work in the evening, and then I'd go out afterward; then I'd sleep until it was time to go out again. Party[ing] and [having] sex were pretty much all that I did, and I had a great time going to the baths and having sex with men, doing a little bit of everything sexually. In Boston at that time, AIDS was not even part of reality.
>
> I drank quite a bit back then. It wasn't a problem or didn't seem to be one. It was fun. I enjoyed it and wouldn't trade those experiences for the world. I did have a couple of relationships, but I wasn't really ready for one at the time, so they never lasted. I wanted to sow my oats, and I didn't need a relationship. Occasionally, I'd go to New York and party and have sex with men there.
>
> Later on, I left Boston and moved to Utah.

Sex and Relationships After AIDS

In 1984, while in Utah, Alexander met a man with whom he would spend the next eight years. AIDS was around then, but AIDS was not, according to Alexander, the reason for his commitment to only one man. In retrospect, he is dissatisfied with his role in that relationship, a relationship in which he appeared to once again take on the role of caretaker, providing his lover with structure, just as he had done as a young adolescent for his sister and father.

Nonetheless, while in the relationship, Alexander practiced monogamy, but he did not speculate on his ex-lover's behavior. Although condoms were not used, Alexander feels he was "safe" from HIV infection, especially as the relationship neared its end and the couple ceased all sexual involvement with each other. Although this may have reduced Alexander's risk of infection, the lack of sex also reduced his quality of life. For Alexander, this negative effect on his quality of life appeared to be related less to his desire for physical pleasure and more to the emotional connections that he associates with sexual intimacy.

> I met Jack in Utah and we moved out here to California together. Our relationship lasted for eight years. We didn't use condoms, but I don't believe that I was at risk for HIV infection. I guess it was a monogamous relationship, but I'm not so sure I want that in my next one. I was monogamous the entire time, but toward the end of that relationship I also did without sex for quite some time.
>
> It wasn't a great relationship. Looking back, I guess it really wasn't a relationship. A relationship for me is when two people are working toward a common goal, to do things together, to work for the future, growing old together. It's affectionate. It's a family.
>
> In this situation, I pretty much enabled my lover. I set the standards and he went along with them. If he needed something, I did it. I always took care of him like I did for my dad after my mother's death. It [the relationship] was based upon what I wanted, and yet I never really got what I wanted. I would decide everything, but what I really wanted was someone to be strong, take the initiative, and, I guess, be the father that I never had. Instead he turned out be a bingeing alcoholic, and he sometimes used drugs. But he somehow kept a job though. It was a relationship in which two people didn't clearly communicate what their needs were.

Eventually he lost interest in sex, so I did without eroticism and lovemaking for a very long—too long of a—time. That was frustrating. I realized that sex is very important to me. Sensuality and eroticism—being intimate, close, and touching someone—are very important to me. Very important.

Sex and Relationships: Today and Tomorrow

Although Alexander is not in pursuit of another lover, he is on the lookout for sexual rendezvous and eroticism. His pending search is a quest for intimacy, not necessarily for "hard and fast" sex. Alexander believes he can achieve intimacy in one encounter and that to do so does not necessarily require an ongoing lover relationship. When I asked him, "What for you is erotic and sensual?" his priorities appeared to be on an emotional plane, or as he called it, an "electrical" plane. Specific sexual acts were of import, but only if they were wrapped in "sexual energy."

> Erotic is intimate, meaning being really in touch with the other person's electricity and energy from a sexual point of a view. I don't have to know the person very well, but I have to tune in. At a certain point, they are directing me to where pleasure exists without telling me where it is. It's being in tune with the other person's pleasure and their being in tune with mine. It's giving and receiving pleasure all at once. It's ecstatic. It's high energy.
>
> Sex is a spiritual act. My spirituality is understanding my inner strength and the energy that allows me to travel through this world. It's energy to be in the world as we see it, and people can connect very well if they're in tune to that energy. I'm a true believer that coincidences are not really coincidences. They happen for a reason. This is related to sexual pleasure because I also feel that my major purpose on this earth is to give pleasure to others as well as to receive it from others. As funny as it sounds, spirituality and sex are about loving people and accepting them as they are.
>
> For physical acts, I am very versatile. I love being oral. Remember, I've always liked licking since I was a child. I like to give head and rimming is always fun. I mostly like to lick and kiss. I find it very exciting.
>
> As far as screwing, I like it but it's not the absolute—*the* sexual experience. During fucking, I don't often do the screwing, but I enjoy it more than getting screwed. I do like ass play though, fingering and

stuff, as long as it's gentle and not too aggressive. Toys, like dildos and vibrators, spice things up too. They're great. But still, these are just acts, ways of reaching pleasure. For me the ultimate goal is giving and receiving pleasurable energy, not performing a specific act.

Since AIDS I have set up boundaries for myself. For example, when it comes to screwing, I use a condom. I do rimming, and sometimes I do get carried away. But I don't think it [rimming] is too much of a risk for HIV infection, but it is for other things like hepatitis. I once worked at an STD [sexually transmitted diseases] clinic, so I am very aware of these kinds of things.

Oral sex, I have it without condoms, and pre-cum doesn't concern me too much. I try to be very aware of what is going on with my mouth. If I have any cuts, tears, or sores, I don't do it. I'm really careful about that. I don't get cum in my mouth, but I miss that a lot.

Alexander yearns to consume his sexual partner's semen, both orally and anally. His necessity for intimacy, not for specific physical acts, may underpin his desire for taking semen within him, a desire to make that "electrical" connection, a connection in which he is taking in his partner's self (Prieur 1990). He explained: "I like taking cum. It is literally being fulfilled, getting something inside of you that belongs to someone else. That's a part of intimacy too, I think."

In keeping with his cravings for intimacy, Alexander described his "perfect sexual partner" by way of emotional, spiritual, and personality characteristics.

I start from a spiritual basis. I prefer someone who is mentally healthy. By that I mean in tune with himself both spiritually and emotionally. That type of person can easily tune into pleasure. Don't get me wrong, I don't want someone who is downright ugly. It's just that physical characteristics are less important, but physical health is also important. Good physical health is also part of being in tune. Oh! And someone who is sexually versatile and willing to play with pleasure.

After I gently pressed him, he moved past his reluctance to provide a physical description of his perfect ideal partner.

I don't have a specific type, but a general rule of thumb is that I'm physically attracted to people who look a lot like me: hairy and dark-skinned types. I find Latino and Greek men to be very attractive, but I was in a relationship with a blond blue-eyed guy for eight years. Go figure."

According to Alexander's earlier testimony, he practices, or at least tries to practice, safer sex. He makes many of the safer sex preparations necessary when he is in the mood to look for a sexual partner. For example, he "usually" discusses condoms and/or his sexual boundaries up-front with a potential sexual partner, and he "usually" keeps condoms and lubricant visually displayed in his bedroom as "a hint."

> Generally, if I am meeting someone, and we start talking, and it's getting really hot, I bring up that I prefer safer sex. I don't like to wait and talk about it in the bedroom. Interestingly, I'm the one who usually brings it up. But anyway, lube and condoms are usually laid out in the bedroom as a subtle hint. Amazingly, a lot of people don't want to use condoms, and that to me is incredible. Hard to believe. If there is any question about using a condom, I insist on it.

However, less than a month before our interview, there was a time when Alexander did not insist that his partner wear a condom. This partner did not fit his favored physical type. Instead he was "very blond, Germanic-looking with blue eyes, and a little younger than" Alexander, but Alexander distinguished the sensual nature of the foreplay and the erotic nature of the sexual encounter as setting this experience apart from his safer sexual experiences. The sensuality of this encounter matched Alexander's notions of "electrical" sexual interaction, his fantasies of connection, and ultimately his ideal sexual pleasure. Because of Alexander's being "tuned into" the sexual pleasure, he felt he could trust this sexual partner even though he did not know the man's HIV status, and unlike his "usual" pattern, safer sex was not discussed prior to embarking upon an "electrical" sexual exploration.

> It was someone I had just met out and about. The sex was wonderful and electrical. It was magical, and I really felt turned on. It was all so very erotic and slow. He was a fabulous kisser, and we were actually using condoms at first. He wanted me to screw him, and then he wanted to screw me. There was a lot of foreplay and we smoked some pot beforehand. I was just into it and so was he.
>
> When he was ready to screw me, he put on a condom but it was too tight for him. So he took it off and screwed me without a condom. I guess it doesn't make a lot of common sense. I guess I thought I could trust him or something since he was so sensual. But it wasn't like I

thought about HIV or anything. I wasn't even thinking about risk. I was into the wonderful electricity. I felt really turned on before I got screwed. It was so very, very pleasurable. It got better and better, and then he came inside of me. I didn't even make him pull out.

As noted in his testimony, Alexander and his partner initially attempted to use a condom, but it was too tight to fit his partner's penis. Alexander's willingness to allow his partner to forgo a condom—though he never expressed it—could be related to his spiritual view of pleasure-giving and pleasure-receiving. After all, a tight condom would surely have reduced his partner's pleasure and thereby Alexander's pleasure. As he took in his partner's semen, Alexander was making a closer connection and thus increasing the intimacy and pleasure that was already spiraling out of control. As Alexander said, "It got better and better." The marijuana may have also added to the synergy by heightening physical sensations (Restak 1994).

Afterward, Alexander pondered his potential risk for HIV infection and analyzed his experience. It was then that he inquired about his partner's HIV status.

I think I'll see this guy again. When I asked him afterwards, he told me he was HIV negative. It's weird that with my lover of eight years, the last time we had sex, it was safe sex. Really strange.

It's human nature to go out and play. Sex really felt better without a condom, but I guess I shouldn't say this since it is so taboo. I've been teaching safer sex for years, telling people how to be prepared, how to discuss safer sex, how to put on condoms, and the works, but it wasn't the risk. It was the pleasure. It's really very humbling to realize that no matter how informed you are, you can take a risk that can be really devastating.

I will get tested in a month or so, and I've done a lot to remain HIV negative. In the last decade, I've preferred monogamy. I always—well almost always—saved my butt [for sex] for the right person. I guess I have remained HIV negative because of timing. I was in a relationship for so long. Partly, too, it [being HIV negative] is due to chance.

Experiences with Death and People Living with AIDS

Beneath a veneer of emotional strength, Alexander has diligently mourned in private and continues to shed tears over his tragic loss of friends and acquaintances whose lives were cut short by HIV. He is, in every sense of the word, a survivor—a survivor who copes with enormous loss by turning to spirituality and therapy.

> I have lost more friends than I can count. I deal with it much differently now than how I used to. In the past, I'd just keep on trucking. Get over it and move on. I did all the lip service of grieving but never really grieved. I finally went to therapy, and through therapy and group recovery work, I got rid of a lot of pain.
>
> I recently had a friend die, and for the first time I was able to be there for him without being consumed by all the others who I have lost. It felt right. Not that it was easy or anything, but with the help of therapy I just felt like I grieved well.
>
> I do ritual too, like in WICCA [a pagan religion]. When a close friend of mine died a while back, I lit incense and burned a candle. I played a song and let him go as the incense went. I think ritual has really helped me deal with grief because it gives me something to do, a way to process it [grief].

In defiance of his loss, Alexander feels "good" about being HIV negative and does not appear to harbor feelings of guilt. In fact, his HIV-negative status gives him a sense of purpose to provide care for and to help those who have become infected. Nonetheless, due to his age of forty-three and his HIV-negative status, Alexander considers himself to be an outsider in the gay community, both in relation to HIV-positive men and to younger HIV-negative men.

> I feel great about being HIV negative. Believe me, I wouldn't want it any other way. I've worked through all that "why not me?" stuff. . . . But I feel like the odd man out sometimes. There's nothing in the gay community directed to HIV-negative gay men my age. We need groups for us, because our experiences are different from younger gay men. We've been around. We came of age [came out] before HIV and have a lot of loss. A tremendous amount. We need to share and connect.
>
> Most of the people that I see in West Hollywood are younger. There aren't many of us older guys left, because so many are dead. There are women around my age, but most of the men have died. And that's a real drag. It's like being a concentration camp survivor when everyone else is gone, but I feel that I am HIV negative for a purpose; and my purpose is to be there for people with HIV, to help them do what they need to do in their lives and for themselves.

Sometimes HIV-positive men feel that I don't understand what it is like to be in their shoes. If they know me well, they recognize that I know what it's like but not what it is to be, but they generally understand that I really care. I am loving and caring. That's my purpose as an HIV-negative gay man, to care for them. That's why I want to stay HIV negative. Somebody needs to care for them, and I am one of those somebodies. That's me.

And that *is* Alexander, a man who despite his shield of age and HIV status will continue to reach out, to care, and to carry on his life-long pattern of providing structure for those in need. Only now, those in need are not his father, sister, or lover, but are sometimes strangers, acquaintances, or friends who are living with AIDS. Following the interview, he headed to work where he would put his own life aside and deal with someone else's crisis, someone with AIDS who needed financial assistance, access to health care, or maybe just someone with whom to talk. As he renders structure to others, however, he cries out for structure of his own, and he strives to make an electrified connection with those like himself: gay men in their forties who are HIV negative—anomalies in West Hollywood today.

6

Roger: Curious Sex

Novelty itself will rivet one's attention. There is a unique moment when one confronts something new and astonishment begins. Whatever it is, it looms brightly, its edges sharp, its details ravishing, in a hard clear light.

—Diane Ackerman, *A Natural History of the Senses* (1990)

O! how this spring of love resembleth, the uncertain glory of an April day, which now shows all the beauty of the sun, and by and by a cloud takes all away.

—William Shakespeare, *Two Gentlemen of Verona*

A waiter-writer originally from Chicago, Roger took notice of a study flyer left at a local coffee shop, a quaint hangout frequented by gays, artists, aspiring actors, writers, and a multitude of what some West Hollywood-ites call "hipster wannabes." Roger arrived at my home on a summer Sunday afternoon, and I met him at the front door with my greeting hand extended. After wiping the sweat from his palm on to his right trouser leg, he rested his burdensome burgundy knapsack at his feet in order to shake my hand. His tall but spare build sported dark knee-length shorts flapping beneath a white tee-shirt, untucked and loose. Sweat pasted his brown bangs to his forehead, and his wire-rimmed glasses had glided down his angular nose, causing him to pause and push them back into place.

I invited Roger to the kitchen where he chose his seat across from me at my kitchen table. While reviewing the informed consent procedure, we both alleviated the stifling heat by downing enormous amounts of water. Roger seemed quite nervous, and his body was stiff with tension. His voice cracked as he responded to the informed consent ritual, and he hesitated, but just momentarily, before assenting. With this formality out of the way, the tape recorder clicked on and we began, slowly at first as Roger rarely ventured beyond curt yes or no answers, due to his diffidence and apparent suspicions. Ultimately, though, he let go of his tension and misgivings by confessing to himself and to me a mystery that he had previously kept concealed.

Childhood

As the youngest child (and only boy, with two older sisters), Roger had firmly fit the profile of "sissy boys" described by Richard Green (1985). Green's sissy boys displayed sex-atypical behaviors during childhood, including a dislike of rough games and sports, a preference for playing with girls rather than with boys, a desire to play with dolls, and a penchant for wanting to wear their mother's or "feminine" clothes. According to Green, boys who held these preferences or who performed these behaviors were more likely to be gay as adults than were other boys.

These sex-atypical behaviors in childhood were a source of stigma for Roger. He grew up in a small Canadian town, and his male peers taunted him because of his "girlie" mannerisms. To cope with this harassment, he attached himself to his older sister (the oldest child), who became his "surrogate mom."

> It seems like I've always felt that I was gay. I remember being attracted to men beginning at an early age. When I was five years old, I wanted to dress up in women's clothes, and come to think of it, I really can't remember any time in my life that I was not attracted to men. I kept a diary just like my sister did, and in my diary I would comment a lot about men who I found attractive.
>
> I grew up in a small town in Canada. It was horrible. Absolutely terrible. I was teased in school from the very first day I started until the day that I graduated. I was teased for being artistic, getting good grades, hanging around with girls in recess, jumping rope, and other "girlie" behaviors. I liked doing those things. I liked doing them a lot. Most of my friends were girls and I liked hanging around with them, but it wasn't like I didn't have any male friends. There were some boys who didn't care what others thought about them, and they would befriend me. I mean . . . I wasn't completely a Carrie. [Carrie is a 1976

movie about a high school girl who is constantly teased and humiliated by her peers for being different. After a particularly cruel incident, she uses her telekinetic powers to lash out in a violent and bloody revenge at her senior prom. Director Brian de Palma's film is a popular cult favorite for some gay men.]

It helped that one of my sisters kept my self-esteem up. My older sister was kind of like my surrogate mom. I was really attached to her, but she died when I was nineteen. My relationship with my living, younger sister was close I guess, but we were always very guarded about our personal lives. And we still are pretty much distant on a personal level.

Roger's parents, both immigrants from Eastern Europe, divorced when he was a small child, but his mother quickly remarried and his father moved away. The emotional distance between Roger as a child and his father may be more related to the father's physical absence than to Roger's sex-atypical behaviors. On the other hand, with his new stepfather, the situation was quite different, and Roger's "not so masculine" behaviors may have played a role in their strained relations.

Although Roger's connection with his mother was more profound, their emotional roles appear inverted. Partly from the turbulent nature of his mother's marriages and partly from the loss of her two daughters (who had left home at an early age), Roger played the role of emotional parent (just as was the case with Alexander in the previous chapter). His mother positioned herself into the role of child and, as one of his "parental" duties, Roger became his mother's confidant.

Growing up, my dad and I were very distant. Since we lived in different countries after my parents' divorce—I was five years old—I only saw him once a year. I really saw so little of him.

My mother and I had a lot of conflict, but it wasn't real heavy conflict as I was a good kid most of the time. . . . I mean . . . I was never into drugs or rebelled in any twisted sort of way. At the same time, I was a caretaker for her because her relationships had turned out to be so horrible.

My relationship with my stepfather stunk. I mean really stunk! Mother married him right after the divorce, and it was really bizarre, because we immediately moved into his house. I literally went from one house to another. My mother married him because she needed to get out of her marriage with my dad. My stepfather gave her a way out in which she could still financially take care of her children. He was actually an old boyfriend, but he never got a chance to really know us. And then presto! Suddenly he was a father. We never liked each other—partly because he was jealous of my relationship with my mom and partly because he knew I was somehow different [given] my not so masculine behaviors. I think it might have been different if I had been an athlete. Our relationship would probably have been less conflict-oriented.

Later on I became my mother's emotional caretaker. She confided in me a lot. I was born late compared to my sisters and they left home early. So that left me and my mom. She always complained to me about things, including about my stepfather.

Coming Out

Although Roger claimed earlier that he feels he has always been gay and attracted to men, he did not come out until he was in his twenties, and his first sexual experience with another man did not occur until he was nineteen and in college.

With the exception of Ralph (Johnny's lover in chapter 2), this makes Roger different from other men in this book. Since Roger came out in the mid-1980s, he belongs to a separate cohort. Unlike previous cohorts of gay men, Roger's cohort came out in the advent of AIDS, at a time when institutions and gay literature provided guidance in the socialization and self-acceptance of young gay men (Gorman 1992; Herdt 1992). Gay literature aided Roger in coming to terms with his behavior and his sexual identity.

> I didn't have my first sexual experience until very late. It was when I was nineteen and in college. I went to college in Chicago and majored in theater, and, you know, theater majors are either gay or at least very gay friendly. There was this very popular guy in the theater department who was attracted to me. Everyone thought he was straight, but little did they know. We became close friends, and he slept over one night. We were just talking and then he suddenly leaned over and kissed me. Just like that. All of a sudden. For me, it was out of the blue, and I had no idea. Things kept going and we had oral sex with each other.
>
> It was all so very exciting and scary at the same time. For me, it was just an experience, but he was in love with me. He idealized me and

wanted to fall in love with another man. I think he was using me as a
catalyst for that, so it didn't really develop into a real relationship.

It was much later that I came out. I read a lot of gay books and stuff,
and when I read the book *Gay Spirit*, my life changed greatly. It helped
me deal with my internalized homophobia and helped in giving me a
good image of gay people instead [of a bad one]. I was twenty-three
when I read it, and I've read it several times since then. It had a real
impact on me and changed my life.

I didn't go out of my way to deny my gay identity by dating girls
or trying to convince others that I was straight, but it took me a while
to come to peace with myself about being a gay man. Rather soon after
I came to feel deep down that I could absolutely say I was gay, I told
my mother. Now our relationship is better than it used to be. Once I
came out, it forced her to confront everything else in her life too. My
mother is an intelligent woman, but she was very shocked at first. She
brought out the Bible and all that kind of stuff, and she cried because
I was a "sinner." When she started going off on me, I told her that her
problems with my being gay were her problems, not mine. She wanted
me to go to therapy, but I told her that she was the one who needed to
go to therapy, not me.

I was really pretty calm about it though. It was a process for her,
and I knew that. Over some time, she did the emotional work that she
needed to do and eventually changed her point of view about gays.
She even recently wrote me a letter telling me that she thought gay
people were some of the few people in the entire world who truly
understand the meaning of the word *integrity*.

For Roger, a gay identity is also a political identity. His politiciza-
tion partially stems from his involvement in the AIDS Coalition to
Unleash Power (ACT UP), where taking action and group identification bolstered his gay identity. Moreover, he feels that sharing this
identity with his mother prompted her to question her own political
worldview as well.

When ACT UP came around, I got involved with the group, and I
learned a lot about AIDS, politics, and my ability to fight for something that I believed in. I went to demonstrations, and I felt really
strong. It was great. Gay was very good to me now.

My mother was very politically conservative at the time. She had a
strong military background and was a Republican. Since she was an
immigrant from Eastern Europe, she was also very anti-Communist in

her political perspective, because it was the communists who killed so many people in our family. After I came out, she began to change. She started watching CNN and C-SPAN a lot and came to realize that her conservative beliefs were not very good. I really feel good about having opened her up to question her staunch political beliefs.

Sex and Relationships: Coming Out in the Time of AIDS

Since Roger belongs to a different cohort than do the older men in this book, he never experienced the "sexual liberation" of the sixties and seventies. This separation is no more clear than in his adult sexual patterns. Roger describes his sexual escapades as "conservative," at least up until the last two years. Roger's individual sexual pattern seems to run counter to the argument of E. Michael Gorman, who, in his 1992 ethnographic account of gay communities in Los Angeles, suggested that there has been a "tempering" of sex and sexuality among gay men because of AIDS. This was undoubtedly the situation in prior years, but in the case of Roger, and the other men in this book as well, it appears that this "tempering" is waning, and that sex and sexuality are once again becoming more central to gay men's lives.

> I've never really had a long-term relationship and in fact I've never really wanted one. I have some intimacy issues that I am currently working on. I find it difficult to connect that closely with another person and, sexually speaking, I've been pretty conservative up until about the last couple of years. I didn't have a lot of one-night stands before, even though I went out to a lot of clubs with my friends. I was mostly just hanging out with friends back then. When I did have sex it was always safer sex. From the media, I knew about HIV as early as 1984, and later on, when I started to identify myself as gay, I got educated about AIDS by my friends, literature put out by agencies, and of course in ACT UP. But the last couple of years has been different for me sexually. I've started enjoying sex a lot more, and I am a little less conservative than I used to be. I have more one-night stands now, and I am enjoying it a lot. That's all. I'm just enjoying it so much, but I still always practice safer sex.

In spite of Roger's avowal of always practicing safer sex—for him safer sex includes oral sex without a condom—he later admitted that his claims of exclusive safer sex were untrue. Even when I asked him,

"When was the last time you had sex that you felt was unsafe?" he told me that he had not had such an experience; but later in the interview, he stopped, apologized, and conceded that he had lied. He lied to me because he was ashamed. He was ashamed of having had anal sex without a condom as the receptive partner less than nine months before the interview. He was also afraid of the humiliation and reactions of gay friends, health educators, and acquaintances if they found out about his behavior.

> For me, safer sex is . . . well . . . oral sex without a condom is a risk that I'm willing to take. . . . I mean . . . life is a risk. After all, my sister was killed in a car accident, and I know nothing is guaranteed. Absolutely nothing. Up until this point in my life, oral sex without a condom is acceptable as long as I am aware of the condition of my mouth. For example, I'm conscious about not having oral sex after flossing my teeth or if something is going on with my gums like bleeding, open cuts, or something.
>
> I tried using condoms for oral sex, but it was just too much to ask. It was denying me something that I didn't want to have denied—to feel the penis in my mouth and touching it with my tongue. To have oral sex without a condom, what's the point? I have heard stories about someone only having oral sex and then seroconverting, but I've never met such a person, so I'm not sure they really exist. Besides, how do I know they are reporting honestly?
>
> Anal sex is different, and I've had it. It's the most dangerous, but I always use condoms when I do it. Always. One time someone tried to fuck me without a condom, and I made them stop and put one on. I don't discuss safer sex up-front. It just happens and is expected. That's why this guy surprised me, but I stopped him.
>
> [*Approximately ten minutes later during a discussion of experiences with people with AIDS*] . . . Stop. I'm really very sorry. Can we go back? I lied to you. This [the interview] is too important. You need to know the truth. . . . This isn't easy, but I gotta tell you that I have had unsafe sex. Only nine months ago. . . . Ashamed . . .[*He looks away from me, turning his head as if he had been slapped*] I can't believe it. Let's go back. This is important and I don't want to mislead you.

Roger's confession raises a couple of important issues about self-reported measures of unsafer sex on closed-ended questionnaires. First of all, questionnaires sometimes ask, "How often do you use a condom?" and offer limited response choices ranging from "never" to "always." In Roger's circumstance, "always" may be an expression of behavior intention (Ajzen 1988), not of actual behavior, thus leading researchers to erroneous interpretations.

Second, Roger is skeptical of the assertions made by individuals who may report oral sex as their only risk behavior for HIV infection. Conceivably this skepticism comes from personal experience as he appears to normally report the same despite behavior to the contrary. Ironically, as I suggested earlier in the introduction, this self-report bias may stem from the success of the gay community's adoption of safer sex as a social norm. Roger is embarrassed by having broken the norm, and thus he is ashamed to admit his transgressions publicly for fear of reprisal; to avoid negative reactions from others, he maintains a public facade of compliance with the norm.

> I'm so surrounded by people who are politically active in AIDS and who are educators about the disease. They make me feel guilty about it when they talk about the risk of infection from fucking without a condom. They get so pompous about it. I have a friend in San Francisco who writes about safer sex. I tried to tell him about my having unsafe sex once, but he believes so strongly that people who could do this [have anal sex without a condom] are screwed up. I'm sure he'd yell at me, so I don't tell anyone. It's embarrassing and I don't want to be ridiculed

So Roger keeps his deviation private and does not share his feelings with friends and acquaintances. As with other gay men who have unsafe sex, he feels alone and wallows in feelings of guilt (see Gold 1995). While speaking about his unsafer experience, Roger's contorted and flushed forehead communicated worry and fear, but once he had finished with his testimony, he fell back into his chair, relieved that he had finally confessed to someone who would not "yell at" him; but he had rushed through the testimonial, not wanting to dwell for too long on such an indelicate topic. Therefore, his description of the event is somewhat sketchy, but nonetheless telling.

Roger had always been curious about anal sex without a condom. Gay men his own age who had come out in their late teens—as well as older gay men—know and have savored the physical sensation of unprotected anal sex. Roger had not, but he had wondered many times what anal sex without a condom would feel like. "It had to feel better," he thought, and he was seduced by his curiosity. In another bit of irony, the prohibitions against anal sex without a condom and the behavior's accompanying risk may have heightened his curiosity as well as his anticipated pleasure (Vance 1984).

I'm totally embarrassed about it. It has troubled me more than I can explain. I've worried and worried a lot. I did get tested for the HIV antibodies three months ago and I'll get tested in another three months just to make sure I'm negative. I didn't even know his [the partner's] HIV status and I never asked him. I was afraid—way too afraid—to ask afterwards.

I met him by way of the computer. Later, we met in person, and I went with him to his apartment. It was purely sexual from the get-go. He was very very very *very*—I can't emphasize it enough—attractive. We had a couple of beers and then we had sex. There was a lot of oral sex beforehand, and I remember that we were pretty worked up. I've been worked up before, but this time was different. I wanted more pleasure and I was curious at some deep level, I guess. I wasn't thinking about AIDS, HIV, or anything. I just didn't stop him when he penetrated me without a condom.

I knew about AIDS when I became sexual, and I have come out with safer sex. I was never into anal sex in my earlier days, but I felt cheated and wanted to experience it [anal sex without a condom] firsthand. I was just always curious about the pleasure of it. It is different than anal sex with a condom. It felt better physically even though I was the one getting screwed and more at risk. That may just have been in my mind, because you're not supposed to think that unsafe sex feels better even if it does. My educator friends say it [thinking condoms are less pleasurable] is a cop-out excuse for unsafe sex. But whatever, it felt great at the time.

Now I know. I'm not curious anymore. I don't think it will happen again. Now I understand why guys say they wish they could fuck the old way, without a condom. It feels warmer and different in you when you are getting fucked without a condom. It's a different physical sensation. . . . Can we talk about something else, now? It's really difficult for me to talk about this.

We did move on. To recount this experience was quite distressing for Roger. He removed his glasses and wiped away apparent tears with the back of his trembling hand, his face radiating a pinkish hue. He apologized for his emotional display, and then his face transformed as he smiled and sighed with relief.

Experiences with Death and People Living with AIDS

Because of his younger age, Roger has not suffered the loss of a great number of friends to AIDS. Still, he has lost one close friend and several casual acquaintances as they grew sicker and sicker until they eventually wasted away.

> I've only known one close friend who died. Most have just been acquaintances. I've visited people in the hospital and stuff. I guess when people die, I pretty much accept it just like I did my sister's death. In a strange way, her death prepared me for the AIDS epidemic. Unlike other people, I guess I knew, even before AIDS, that being young did not equal living forever. And my spiritual beliefs aren't final, and so I guess that I accept death. I'm sad when someone dies, but I don't think to myself that their death is an injustice. Death is a natural part of living.

Roger's references to his sister's death continued throughout the interview as we discussed issues of death and dying. On the one hand, her death contributes to his ability to cope, but on the other, it induces impatience and frustration with people who have HIV and do not accept death as he has accepted it.

> I know someone who has end-stage AIDS. He's not a real close friend. I just help him out sometimes because I am a nice guy. He does not live a healthy life. I know he has a lot of issues right now, but part of me wants to say, "you know what? My sister was killed in a car accident without living her whole life. You're older than she was when she died. Yeah, you feel hopeless, and yes, I can't imagine what you're going through; but you've lived more of a life than my sister. You have to accept it. It is what it is."

Roger may have gone too far in his acceptance of death. Out of all the men I interviewed, he was the only one who fell into a class of gay men who harbor feelings that they will not survive the epidemic even though they are currently HIV negative (Odets 1995).

> If I were positive, I guess I could stop worrying about things like seroconverting. After I get tested, I never feel like I've made it. I'm never home free. I'm just OK at this point in time, but since I'll never just dry kiss a sexual partner or give them massages, I could, I guess, potentially get infected.

Odets argues that this belief of inevitable infection can and does lead to unsafe sexual experiences, but to make such a suggestion in this case requires an interpretive jump that excludes the situations (i.e., curiosity about pleasure and an attractive partner) surrounding Roger's sexual experience. After all, Roger does not always and did not always have sex without a condom. Besides, as I argued earlier in chapter 1, it is just as likely that such feelings stem from the unsafer experience instead of, or in addition to, being a causal factor for unsafer sex. Roger's terminal belief may, however, drive him to persistent HIV testing.

> I worry about sex without a condom, even oral sex. Sometimes I worry so much that I go to get tested at my doctor's office instead of at an anonymous test site. That way I don't have to wait for two weeks to get my results. I never know for sure what the test will say, so I don't want to sweat out a long wait.

Before the interview came to an end and Roger departed, he sat in silence as if another thought, something unsaid, was concealed beneath his tongue. I asked him if he had something else he wanted to say. He suspended his thoughts briefly before giving a muttered response of "no." Then without revealing another detail, he took another long drink of water and headed for the door. I will never know what else he may have wanted to share, but as I watched him walk away through my front gate, his tall back seemed less hunched and his chin raised an inch or so higher. I can only hope that, having shared his "dirty little secret," his emotional burden is a little less cumbersome.

7

Jerry: Leather Sex

I think it's very hot to see someone in film who's obviously enjoying some particular fetish, if you think they're really digging it, I think it turns you on.

—Fred Halstead, "An Interview with Fred Halstead" (1979)

What is erotic? The acrobatic play of the imagination. The sea of memories in which we bathe. The way we caress and worship things with our eyes. Our willingness to be stirred by the sight of the voluptuous. What is erotic is our passion for the liveliness of life.

—Diane Ackerman, *A Natural History of Love* (1994)

Thirty-eight-year-old Jerry telephoned me in late May 1994, one week after I had interviewed one of his friends, who informed him of the study—and of the twenty-five-dollar dispensation for each interview. Jerry figured that participating in the study "would be an easy way to pick up some bucks." He elected that I interview him at my home because, as he matter of factly told me in a deep, almost hoarse-sounding voice, his apartment was "a total mess."

When he arrived that Saturday morning, he wore an old pair of gray sweat pants, and his blond thatch of hair was disheveled. Neatness did not appear to be a significant virtue to Jerry, at least on his day off from work. Instead he strove for comfort. For his interview, he chose the living room sofa, complete with large, fluffy pillows, forgoing the hard-backed wooden chairs at my kitchen table. He maintained a relaxed posture throughout, slouching back into the plushy sofa and only once raising himself up to lean forward.

Childhood

Unlike Roger, Jerry was never a "sissy boy" and did not exhibit sex-atypical behaviors. He played with "Tonka trucks and building blocks" and was, much to his father's delight, a pitcher for a Little League baseball team. Jerry grew up in a small North Carolina town buried in the Pisgah National Forest, not far from the Blue Ridge Parkway. The town's population was just a few thousand, a place where, Jerry said, "Men were men and women were women." Deer hunting was a fall and winter passion, and Jerry passed many a frigid day with his father, gun in hand, patiently awaiting the bushy bob of a leaping stag.

Jerry was an only child, and both his mother and father were attentive to his wants and needs. His relationship with his father was the pillar of his childhood, a relationship that Jerry feels contributed to his masculinity and to his emotional stability.

> I was an only child and we lived in the country. There weren't many other kids around to play with. I joined Little League, which was a godsend. If it hadn't been for Little League, I would have been a loner—at least during the summer when school was out. My mother would always take me wherever I needed to go, and she would wait in the car or gossip with the other moms while I was at ball practice. Both my mom and dad encouraged me to succeed and did all that they possibly could do to make sure that I did [succeed]. I never felt rejected by my father like some of my other gay friends.
>
> I had lots of friends at school and in Little League. I guess you could say I was very popular. Our family had lived in the area for a long time and we were well known throughout the county. We lived in my grandfather's house after he died, and people would always refer to the house by our last name—the Wilkes' Place.
>
> I wasn't your stereotypical homosexual kid. I played with boys' toys like Tonka trucks, baseballs, and footballs. I got excited over baseball mitts, not over Barbie dolls. There's nothing wrong with guys playing with dolls. I'm not one of those guys who hates queeny [effeminate] men, but it just wasn't me. . . .
>
> My father was very important to me. We spent a great deal of time doing father and son things, and I will always appreciate that very much. He came to all my baseball games and cheered along with my

mom every time we won a game, and he always tried to make me feel better after we lost a game. I was very fortunate. I hear horror stories about other gay men and their childhoods and how it has fucked them up, but mine was great. No abuse from family or peers. I just a had a stable environment. . . . Thank God.

Dad used to take me hunting with him. Hunting was a big to-do in North Carolina. It was what men did and only men. They [men] would get together, sneak a bottle of whiskey under the truck seat or in the glove compartment, and head out to the woods and wait. The waiting and the cold weather could sometimes be miserable, but I was always glad to go along with my father. I had my own gun by the time I was eight years old, and my father taught me how to use it. He was a great father.

We went to church most Sundays, but my parents weren't religious fanatics. I have to say that because everyone always thinks if you're southern and Christian, then you must be a fanatic. My parents both believed strongly in God, and I was taught a literal interpretation of the Bible; but at home, they didn't preach and pray all the time. Religion was just a normal part of our lives.

As a young boy, Jerry participated in sexual play with some of the Little League team members, but these experiences never elicited an emotional response from him. For Jerry it was "just play." However, when Jerry was thirteen, he became infatuated with one of his father's hunting buddies. This man represents Jerry's first memories of emotional desire for another male and, as will be demonstrated later in his testimony, this man also represents the perfect male physical type about which Jerry would fantasize for the rest of his life.

You know how little boys can be. My Little League friends and I would talk about girls, especially older girls with breasts, and show each other our little weenies, as if we were big men. It was just play. There was one guy on the team who I would consider my best friend. Jimmy slept over at my house and I sometimes slept over at his. Our parents were good friends too.

On one of those sleep-overs—I was about ten or eleven, I think— Jimmy brought over a *Playboy* magazine. He said his older brother got it for him in Asheville. We looked through it while we were lying in bed, and we talked a lot about sex: why sex with girls, of course. The women all had big boobs, and it was the first time I had ever seen a vagina. Neither one of us really knew much about it, but I remember getting a hard-on, pulling off my underwear, and playing with myself. I moved closer to Jimmy and the head of my penis was touching him. He reached down and made some comment about his being bigger than mine. I asked him to prove it and he did. It was bigger, and I assumed it was because Jimmy was one year older than me. I remember my heart beating real fast when I reached out and touched his penis. It was all happening so fast that I guess I was real nervous about it. He touched mine and we started rubbing up against one another, and we beat off together. I guess that was my first sexual experience. Jimmy and I would sometimes teach other boys how to masturbate. We never thought it was a bad or evil thing to do—I guess because we always talked about girls while doing it, and masturbation was never talked about in Sunday school as either good or bad. It just wasn't talked about at all.

The first time I got a real feeling of attraction to another man was when I was around thirteen years old. My father had a hunting buddy named Steve. Steve was in his twenties and married to one of the teachers at my school. He was really handsome with blond hair, a red beard, and blond hair on his chest. He wasn't muscular, but he was naturally stocky. I mean he didn't go to a gym or anything, he just had a naturally big build. I remember I'd stare at him a lot and I'd get a warm feeling all over. I began to fantasize about him when I masturbated, and anytime we went hunting I would always ask my father if Steve was coming along. I still didn't know what this was about.

On one of our hunting trips, I was stationed alone with Steve while my father was further down the way. Well, when you're outside and have to pee, there is only one place to go, and Steve turned around and was peeing. I got up. I don't know what came over me, but I saw his penis. It was bigger than mine too. I remember touching it, and he jumped. He pushed my hand away. When he was done peeing, he winked at me and said something like "yours will be big too when you get to be a man." I was shaking all over, but he was really nice about it. I mean, he could've yelled at me or told my father, but he never mentioned it; and I never tried to touch him again. But I still fantasized about him.

Jerry does not recollect having another sexual or presexual encounter with a man until he was seventeen. In the meantime, he dated girls, and at one point he became "pre-engaged" to a cheer-leader named Cindy. Cindy was his first and only sexual relation with a female, and he tells about this event as if it served as a rite of passage into manhood.

I was a football player in high school, and of course I was popular with the girls, especially the cheerleader bimbo types. I dated girls when I was sixteen after I got my driver's license and my first car. I'd take girls to the drive-in movies a lot. I knew that many of my friends were experimenting sexually and I was still—for all practical purposes—a virgin. I hadn't screwed a girl yet. And me a football player! There was a lot of pressure for jocks to lose their virginity.

I had a steady girl named Cindy. Of course she was a cheerleader, and got around a lot. I was determined to screw her so that I could finally talk about my experience with the other jocks. I had to screw her or the other guys would think I was gay. I knew what gay was at this time, but I didn't—or I guess I didn't want to—think that I was or even could be gay. I was just a jock wanting to make it with a girl to prove his manliness. Looking back, it seems really silly.

One Saturday night Cindy and I went to see a movie at the drive-in. Everybody who was dating would go there first and then to a place out in the country where we could neck and smooch. There were plenty of private places in the country. At the drive-in, I slipped my hand beneath Cindy's dress. She smiled because she wanted this too. She was a cheerleader, and I knew that most of them were not virgins. I think she wanted to get married to me, and we were already pre-engaged. Now that was a stupid thing: getting pre-engaged. [*I ask him to explain*] I guess it just meant that we would probably get engaged and married one day. It was a step above going steady. When I slipped my hand beneath her dress, I think she scooted up so that I could get into her panties. I just remember she was very, very willing. I fingered her and, for some reason, I'm not sure why, but I knew that I was not the first boy to go there. She put her hand on my crotch and I had a hard-on. Later we drove out to the country and I screwed her. There wasn't much to it. It felt good I guess, but I remember it wasn't nearly as good as all the other guys told me it would be. I was sort of disappointed, but anyway, I was a man now. I had finally screwed a girl, but with no condom, mind you. I'm lucky she didn't get pregnant. We broke up soon afterward because I just wasn't interested anymore. . . .

Later on, when I was about seventeen, I had sex—just oral sex—with another guy. This was one of my football buddies. We used to drive around town together in his Mustang—you know, the usual obnoxious high school boy thing: yelling at girls, drinking beer, driving fast, acting stupid. One night we were pretty drunk and pulled the Mustang over to the side of the highway. I was afraid we were going to have an accident. He started talking about how he wished he had a girl to fuck and how he was so horny. He pulled his cock out and started masturbating, and I did the same. I remember staring at his cock and it was the "I'll suck yours if you'll suck mine" routine. And we did. [*I ask him how he felt about it afterward*] We never talked about it afterward. We pretended that it hadn't happened, and I felt sort of dirty the next day; but I also felt great because I knew that I enjoyed that much better than the time I screwed Cindy. It was then that I figured out that something was going on and I wasn't just some horny jock.

Coming Out

After graduating from high school in 1974, Jerry attended college in Atlanta with plans to go on to medical school. He found a small bachelor apartment in the midtown area of Atlanta, but he did not know beforehand that Atlanta's midtown area is one of the city's centers of gay activity. In his new milieu, Jerry expeditiously confronted and embraced his sexuality, plunging himself exclusively into a gay culture, leaving the heterosexual world behind. It was not that he devalued the heterosexual world (see Cass 1979), but he was so involved with other gay men and sexual adventure that he had little time left over for making and maintaining heterosexual relations and friendships.

I was lucky. When I took my apartment, I had no idea that the building was primarily a gay building. Well . . . maybe that's not completely true. I thought something was up when I first looked at the place and the landlord was eyeing me, but I just pushed it to the back of my mind.

I quickly made friends with one of the gay guys in the building. Well . . . he seduced me. He was a butch clone and wore construction worker garb all the time—plaid shirts, jeans, work boots—blond of course, as I like them, and a rather big hunky guy. He was the first person I ever fucked, and I knew from that moment on that being a top was my calling. This was around 1975 or 1976. He showed me a lot of fun things and introduced me to the bookstores that would set me on the path of ill repute. [Some gay bookstores are business establish-ments where pornographic magazines, videos, and other items are sold in the front, while in the back there are areas for men to cruise and have sex.] I liked those places. Eventually, I'd meet one or more guys and go into one of the rooms off the hallway where for a quarter you could put on a porno flick and have sex. If you let the movie stop, they had guys who would pound on the door and tell you to put more money in or get out. Sometimes I'd go in and put on porno and watch through glory holes [holes in the wall] the guys making out in the booth next door or stick my cock through the hole for them to play with. It was something. I got into it, and I started getting more into the leather scene. I went to a place called Mrs. Peas—I think that was the name of the place. It was a bar that had a back area for cruising and sex. I started drinking a lot and did crystal speed [methamphetamine] and MDA [a hallucinogenic] occasionally to make the sex more excit-ing. It was so strange, but that was what a lot of us did back then. I don't have no regrets about any of it. I enjoyed it tremendously and am glad to have those memories.

During all this time, I started coming out. I became a clone with a mustache, short hair, jeans, and wore keys hooked on a belt loop on my left side to signal that I liked to fuck. I became very sexual, but I still didn't tell people about being gay. They could probably tell any-way by the way I dressed. I exclusively hung out with gay people for the most part, not because I didn't like heterosexuals or anything like that, just that between school and my nightlife I had little time for making friends outside of my gay group, so I guess it really wasn't like I had anyone to come out to. I had left most of my high school friends behind in North Carolina, and when I went home for visits I rarely saw them. They were all married, and most of the girls were already pregnant. When I did visit old school friends, I didn't talk about being gay. I avoided them or else I would talk about girls around them.

Jerry still has not come out to his parents or to his high school friends. Given the geographical distance that separates him from them, Jerry sees little need to share his identity. Moreover, he feels that his relationship with his mother and his father does not suffer from the secrecy.

My parents. My parents still do not know. They are in North Carolina and I am here. There's really no need to tell them. I rarely go home and they don't visit here. I speak with my father a lot and we talk about work, the weather, hunting season, and sports. It doesn't bother me that he and mother don't know that I am gay. My relationship with my father is very good from a distance, and I'd like to keep it that way. I am still close with him and we can talk about so many other things, but I'm sure he would have a negative reaction to my being gay; but because of his old age, I shouldn't expect him to change. Old people don't change their ways so easily. Neither of us needs the grief.

It really isn't a big burden or anything like that. When I had a lover, we went home to visit a couple of times. Both my mother and father were nice to both of us, but we slept in separate rooms. Jack [the lover] hated it, but I didn't mind. It is their house after all, and I think they truly believed that we were just friends. Why burst their bubble? I personally think it would be selfish of me to do so. They have their feelings, and they aren't interfering in my life for the most part. Some of my friends call me closeted, but I don't need people to tell me that I'm OK so that I can feel OK.

While attending school in Atlanta, Jerry eventually switched over to the university's nursing program because it was a faster track than continuing on to medical school. His father was not thrilled about this change in direction, as he wanted a doctor in the family, but he continued to support, both emotionally and financially, Jerry's education.

In spite of Jerry's earlier claim of having "no regrets" for his actions, he qualified this later on in his second interview. Today Jerry does regret that he did not continue on to medical school and blames his "gay life overload" for interfering with his life goal of becoming a doctor. Although whether or not an active gay life in the 1970s had a negative impact on most gay men's ability to achieve life goals is a matter of debate (see McWhirter and Mattison 1984; Murray 1992), Jerry does feel that his gay "fast life" of bars and back rooms caused him to compromise his career aspirations.

> I changed my major to nursing so that I wouldn't have to continue on into medical school before getting a job and becoming financially independent. Besides, I wanted to play and explore my sexuality and not be tied down to studying for long hours. Medical school and play don't fit together. I wanted to go to work, come home, and then go out, party, and have sex. I wish I had gone to medical school now, but what's behind me I can't change. Besides, I'm doing pretty well financially and I like my work.

I remember that my changing over [to nursing] pissed my father off. He really wanted me to be a doctor, and you know nursing is thought of as a woman's profession. I think he still tells people that I am a doctor or something instead of admitting that I am just a nurse. He believes that boys should do boy things and girls should do girl things and the two should never cross. But he continued to pay for my education and encouraged me to stay in school. He didn't disown me.

Sex and Relationships Before AIDS

Throughout the 1970s and early 1980s, Jerry continued his sexual exploits, ultimately developing a fetish for leather. Although leather is an essential element of his erotic desires, he does not define himself as a sadist or masochist as he does not administer to or receive high levels of pain from a sexual partner. He limits his delivery of painful sensations to "mild" spanking, using his hand or a leather accoutrement, on his partner's buttocks.

Jerry also acquired a sexual appetite to dominate his partner, and anal penetration as the inserter provides him with an erotic sense of domination (see Davies et al. 1993). He chooses to be in control of a given sexual situation, but within limits. He does not want, in his words, a "sex slave, someone who lets me completely dominate them. I like a little resistance. I just like being the man." Being the man means being the penetrator.

Some research suggests that Jerry's preference for being the insertive partner may in fact be related to his "conventional" (meaning supposedly like a heterosexual male's) childhood in which there appears to have been little, if any, sex-atypical behaviors. Namely, the argument goes, the desire for primarily being an insertive partner or receptive partner in anal sex is a continuation of a lifelong form of sexual expression of more masculine behaviors or more effeminate ones (LeVay 1994).

This may be correct, but there is at least one other factor at play: pain. For example, Jerry insists, as do many other men who prefer to penetrate rather than to be penetrated anally (see Davies et al. 1993), that he simply finds anal sex as a receiver to be too painful.

The seventies and even the eighties were fantastic for being a gay man. There was lots of sex. It was easy to find, and you didn't have to worry about incurable viruses and bacteria wandering about. Just get a shot, pop a pill, or what not—and poof!—no more little bug. It was all so easy.

I really got into the leather scene, but not into S&M [sado-masochism]. That was too much for me. The kinkiest thing I ever did was when I was on acid once, and I made this guy drink my urine. I only did that once, and that was my limit. I never wanted to pull around a slave on a leash or hurt people too much, just a little spanking and maybe make them lick my boots. I never wanted a sex slave, someone who lets me completely dominate them. I like a little resistance. I just like being the man.

I really do like leather. I know that sounds a little kinky, but probably not to you as you're gay too. [*I nod*] Leather smells manly, and it turns me on like nothing else can. I like having sex while just wearing a leather vest or chaps or something leather. I've just about always kept a leather whip, but I never hit anyone too hard, just enough to leave a little red mark on their butt. When I'm fucking someone, I spank them. I like it rough, but not all that piercing and injury-causing stuff. . . .

I learned all of this—about what I like—because of the sexual freedom of the times. I was able to find out what turns me on and now I know it and can experience the fun. I also discovered some things I didn't like. [For example,] I don't like to be fucked because I don't like the way it feels. I tried it once and the guy had a big penis, and it hurt way too much. I guess the guys I fuck don't feel pain. I don't know why that is. Maybe they just get a lot of practice at it.

On a good weekend [back in the seventies], I used to have sex with maybe three or four guys, but usually one or two. I never liked to see the same guy for too long. I would date someone for a week or two. Maybe. But I preferred going out to the back rooms and to orgies where men could experience something new all the time. I was exploring my sexual side.

All I can say is that it was great. There were no worries, just a lot of fun and sex. It was like I had left the old me, the perfect son and football player, back in North Carolina. I guess I just let loose all that stored-up sexual energy. I would do anything to bring those good old days back. Anything.

As far as relationships, I never wanted one back then. It would have been a ball and chain for me because I wasn't ready for commitment.

I still feel that way. I didn't have a lover relationship until 1986, and it didn't last for more than a year.

Sex and Relationships After AIDS

In 1981 Jerry moved to West Hollywood, accepting a nursing position with a doctor's office that served both a heterosexual and homosexual clientele. Thus he witnessed some of the first cases of AIDS at a time when its etiology was not yet known.

> I remember how afraid everyone was when AIDS came along. I saw it at the doctor's office where I worked, and I must admit I was afraid too. We didn't know how it was transmitted, but I always thought it was sexually transmitted, probably because it was mostly gay men coming down with it. But we figured it might be more than one disease since people showed up with pneumonia and Kaposi's sarcoma [KS]. A lot of the people in LA that I had sex with would eventually die and some of my friends back in Atlanta too.
>
> I was relieved when we finally got the antibody test. I know a lot of people didn't want to take it because they were thinking, "Well, if I have HIV, I can't do anything about it because there is no treatment, and so why bother?" I bothered. I thought I wanted to know. I wanted to plan my life if necessary and decide what I would do with the time I had left. I got tested in 1987, and I started using condoms after that and educating other people—I guess because I worked at the doctor's office and saw people who were sick.

In 1986, out of fear of AIDS and in response to the educational messages of the time urging gay men to reduce their number of sexual partners, Jerry found a lover and settled down, if only for a short period of time, into a relationship masked with a monogamous front. But Jerry would not be content with spending his life with just one sexual partner and sought out other men to alleviate his sexual boredom.

> I thought I would have to get into a relationship to keep from getting infected. We kept being told, "reduce your number of sex partners." So I did . . . well . . . sort of. I got into a relationship with Jack. He was a sweet and very handsome guy: blond, blue-eyed, masculine, and a successful business professional. We promised each other that we

would be monogamous, but even though he was a perfect man and incredibly good-looking, I couldn't do it.

He was good in bed too. We didn't use condoms. I think we were in denial or something, and we were in love, or at least he was. Of course, sex feels better without a condom, and we thought that by being monogamous—even though I wasn't—we wouldn't be at risk if we were infected, and if we were . . . well . . . it wouldn't matter anyway. I didn't get tested until 1987, but Jack never got tested until he came down with pneumocystis carinii pneumonia [an HIV-related opportunistic infection] in 1989. By then we had broken up, but I was devastated and immediately went to see him. I held his hand throughout, and we both wondered how I had not gotten infected. With my behaviors, I was the more likely candidate—except that he was a bottom and I was a top. It was really weird. We were only together a year and probably would have stayed together if I had kept my zipper zipped, but again I just couldn't commit sexually to just one man. Emotionally, I loved Jack with all my heart. He was a sweet man, and I wish that I had treated him better.

I tried to be monogamous but I couldn't. We lived in West Hollywood, and Jack traveled a good bit. Sometimes I would walk down La Jolla [a street where gay men cruise] and see a hot guy. I couldn't resist it. I only cheated on him three times in our year together. He finally figured it out and left me. He felt that I had betrayed him. For him sexual fidelity was love. He finally found a monogamous partner who also stood by him until he died. We remained friends and it was difficult to let him go.

After his relationship with Jack ended, Jerry resumed his favorite sexual behaviors though their frequency was diminished by the specter of the AIDS epidemic. He also acquired an additional change in his sexual repertoire—using condoms, at least most of the time—and added a new twist as well: more extensive acting out of leather fantasies.

Once I was a free man, I went wild again, but nothing like in the seventies. I used a condom or at least tried to most of the time. Condoms are not too great to use. The packages are a bitch to get open sometimes. I mean, here I am looking sexy, trying to be smooth, and fumbling with the package. It's sort of like making a move on someone, and then you realize that you've got something like spaghetti sauce on your chin the whole time. I know you're supposed to practice and, believe me, I've had a lot of practice, but it's still interrupts the sexual flow.

I use condoms. I really do. Sometimes—but it really doesn't happen much—the sex [gets] too hot and I forget about a condom. I know that sounds terrible, but I am a human after all. People forget that sometimes, that gay men are human like everybody else. Straight men go looking for sex, and everyone looks the other way. Nobody says doodlie-squat. Straight people have a lot of unsafe sex. That is how women get pregnant, unless everyone's using turkey basters [artificial insemination]. Don't they [heterosexuals] understand that? [*I shrug*]

. . . I don't think that I thought much about it [not using a condom]. It wasn't like I was playing around and thought, "This is great. Forget the condom. I don't want to bother." It would just happen.

For oral sex, no way! I never have and never will use a condom. They taste horrible and the risk of infection is low. It's like sucking on a tire. I don't know anyone who uses those things for sucking. . . .

To keep the sex safer and not boring, I started getting more into my leather thing and acting out fantasies while using a condom, just like they teach in those workshops. [*I ask him to describe one of his fantasies*] My favorite fantasy is to tie the guy up while he lays naked, face down on the bed. I use leather, of course. I like to have a lot of leather things like chaps, vests, caps, and boots scattered around the room. Then I like to lick him [the sexual partner] all over, have him chew on pieces of leather and beg to be fucked, and I especially like the begging part. I don't know why it excites me so much, but it does. It's great and then I'll end it by putting on a condom and fucking him. I started making the sex act last longer by playing around more beforehand. I still like these kinds of fantasies, and I am very happy that I can keep my sex fun and enjoyable regardless of HIV. It's not sex that puts you at risk. It's unsafe sex. I do the best that I can to enjoy sex. It's important to me. It's an important part of my life, and anyone, straight or gay, who says it does not play an important role in theirs is lying and not being honest with themselves or with anybody else.

Sex Today and Tomorrow

In his above testimony, Jerry says that sometimes the sex gets "too hot," and when it does, he does not use a condom. This has happened approximately three times in the last three years. I asked him to define what he means by "too hot," and his explanation was based upon his partner's physical attributes in relation to the attributes of his ideal partner, and the erotic context of the sex act in relation to his ideal fantasy.

Given this, it may be that implementing the safer sex message of "act out your fantasies" could have an opposite impact than that desired by educators. In other words, acting out his "hottest" fantasy may play a role in increasing the probability that Jerry will not use a condom (see Gold et al. 1991). To further explore this possibility, I asked Jerry to identify any differences between his last sexual encounter without a condom with his general safer sexual experiences, and then to describe for me any and all details he could recall about the former.

> That [when he had sex without a condom] was totally different. In an odd way it was perfect. Absolute perfection . . . until the next day. There was lots of leather and action. We were all over the place, and he was definitely my type. I couldn't have placed a more perfect order. I'm not sure what happened, but we both just got into it.
>
> It was October, about a week before Halloween [approximately eight months before the interview]. I had made a date that night with a guy I had been seeing for about a month, but it wasn't anything too serious. We were just dating, but he bagged out on me, and so I got leathered-up in my chaps and vest and went down to the Spike [a West Hollywood Levi's/leather bar]. I was hanging out and talking with some friends of mine. I had a couple of beers, and then this guy came by me, cruising me real heavy-like. I mean it was one of those times when you know that he definitely wants it.
>
> He stopped and stood against the wall not too far away from me. He was gorgeous: big, blond, blue-eyed, red goatee, and an athletic build. He looked very Nordic, and he had on jeans and a leather vest, no shirt. His chest had reddish-golden hair. I just wanted to reach out and pull it. We kept staring at one another while my friends kept talking away. I don't remember what we were talking about, but they kind of caught on to the fact that I was cruising, so they said goodbye and wandered around the bar. The guy immediately came over and we talked for a while. I don't remember what about, but he did tell me that he was from New York and was visiting friends here. One thing led to another and we went to my place. Luckily, I had cleaned the place up a little bit since I was expecting a date. And my room was ready for some play. The lube was out. Leather was out. Condoms were on the nightstand next to some towels for cleaning up afterwards.

As soon as we got to my condo, we got started kissing and groping. It was unbelievable. Truly unbelievable. He was just aggressive enough and submitted to my directions. He bit at my nipples through my leather vest, and it was obvious that we had leather in common. We eventually got undressed, except I kept my leather vest on, and we were both wearing leather cockrings with snaps. His cock was huge. Maybe my memory is exaggerating it a bit, but I swear it must have been eleven inches. Not that I have to have a big penis. I'm not really a size queen, but I do enjoy oral sex more if the guy is hung.

He turned out to be a bottom. He let me take complete charge. We played in the living room, mostly oral sex. He sucked me and, given the size of his penis, I definitely sucked him. It started getting a little wild, and I would pound his chest a little and pinch at his nipples.

We went into the bedroom. All my leather stuff in the room seemed to really turn him on. I pushed him on the bed and fell on top of him. He was a perfect man to dominate: strong and Nordic. We continued on with oral sex. I put tit clamps on his nipples, which were already calloused and stretched from use, and so I knew he would like that. I pulled on them, and I was right. He loved it. Then I'm not sure how it came up, but I used strips of leather and tied him [his wrists] to my bedposts, face down. He started begging me to screw him. It was incredible, I tell you. I spanked him with my hand, not real hard, but made some red marks on his butt. He kept begging, and I kept encouraging him by saying things like, "Do you want it?" He really seemed to [want it].

At first, I rimmed his butt. It was great and well-shaped with dimples on each cheek. He was shaven around the anus, so it was all pretty clean. I had his body very well greased with Wet [a popular lubricant] and started fingering him. I gave him some poppers [amyl nitrate] at this point. The poppers were on the nightstand beside the condoms, but when I reached for the bottle, I don't remember seeing them. Then I don't know, I just slipped in. For a second, I guess I thought about a condom. They were on the nightstand, but I didn't stop and he just kept screaming, "Yeah, don't stop!" I guess I didn't stop. That sounds dumb, doesn't it? I mean saying, "I guess I didn't stop." I didn't stop. Plain and simple.

While I was going on with screwing, he was chewing a leather glove that I wore on my right hand and had used to finger him with. It went on for a long time. I would stop and he would beg for more. It was incredible. I know I keep saying that, but it *was* incredible. Then, I don't know—I feel real crummy about this now—but I didn't even pull out. It was like being possessed. I just came inside of him. Then I untied him. I still didn't feel bad about it yet, and I jerked him off.

We didn't say a lot afterward, but fell asleep. The next morning, we had sex again. This time I put on a condom and the sex was more gentle. I apologized for not wearing one the night before, and he asked me my HIV status. I told him I was negative, and he was too. I felt horrible. I couldn't believe what I had done. I just couldn't believe it. It had only happened a couple of times before since my relationship, and I had sworn it would not happen again, but it did. I felt ashamed and dirty. Very, very ashamed and dirty.

About six months before this encounter, Jerry had a somewhat similar experience. The partner had many physical similarities to the one described above. Jerry met this other partner at the same bar and the sexual dance matched Jerry's fantasy. Again he skipped the condom.

Prior to that, it's difficult to remember. That time the guy was blond again, really tight build. Somewhat slimmer than the other guy. . . . I met him at the Spike, and I had had a couple of beers and was laughing. Having a good time. I picked him up and brought him back to my place. [*I ask him what the partner was wearing*] Oh yeah, he was wearing leather too, just a vest and leather boots, I think. It was crazy like the other time. We were all over the place, and he let me dominate him. He did everything I wanted him to do. I asked him to bend over so that I could ass play a little, which I did with my leather glove, and I just put it [his penis] in and he didn't stop me. I don't remember if I was thinking about it much. I'm not sure, but I don't believe so. I was just into it, going for the gold as far as I can remember. I don't remember thinking about anything.

Less than a week before the interview, Jerry had also had a safer sex experience. The description of this event is remarkably different from his unsafer encounters. This time the sex was "great" but not as "hot" or zestful. He met the safer partner at a different type of gay bar, and the partner's physical appearance and sexual role are not the same as they were for Jerry's unsafer episodes.

He was a younger guy, brownish hair with not much on his chest, who loved oral sex. So that was mostly what we did. I met him at the Gold Coast [a neighborhood gay bar]. I was out with friends again, sipping on some brews. He came to my place, but he really wasn't into the leather scene too much. He liked his nipples pinched, but not much more rough-housing than that. I did screw him with a condom. It's weird, I guess. I just reached over, like on automatic, and put the condom on—not like the other times I talked about [the unsafer experiences]. It's not that I thought they [the other men] were safer or nothin', just . . . I'm not sure. I was into the sex this time, but I didn't just stick it in like with the other guys. It was great sex but not too wild. He wanted a daddy so I played with him some, but domination is more than being a daddy. I like dominating an equal, not a son figure. We were only doing it for about half an hour to forty-five minutes or so. He left and I haven't seen him since. Like I said, it was great sex, but not the best in the world.

It appears rather evident then that Jerry is quite capable of practicing safer sex—and he knows it—but an unsafe encounter can still occur. Likewise, he still feels shame and guilt after having taken a sexual risk. Following one of Jerry's unprotected sexual escapades, he confided in another nurse at his office who he though might be sympathetic. Instead, the female nurse "went ballistic." She accused Jerry of not caring about himself and of being suicidal. Because of her response, he confided in no one the next time he did not wear a condom, and he would only tell me about his experience because he could do so while using an alias. He also wanted me to promise "not to lecture" him, a promise I readily gave and kept.

Jerry tested negative again in March 1994, six months following his last slip, and he wishes to remain negative. Although he has given it much thought, he still cannot understand why he took such a risk. He only knows that he was so enthralled in his sexual encounter that he just didn't use a condom. Despite this, his intention to continue practicing safer sex is high; but his belief that he can maintain safer sex has been somewhat—though only slightly at this point—damaged by his occasional slips (Ajzen 1988; Bandura 1986).

> The time before when I had had unsafe sex, I tried to tell this woman at work. She was a friend of mine. I thought she would understand my predicament since I knew that she'd had unsafe sex with her boyfriends and was worried sometimes. But when it came to me, she went ballistic like a real zealous bitch. She started screaming at me, telling me that I was fucking with my life. She even called me suicidal. Boy, how that didn't help my situation. I felt even worse, and I felt like a

fool. This last time I didn't use a condom, I didn't tell her or anyone else. I didn't want to hear it, not from anyone. I was beating my own head into the wall. I didn't need anyone else whacking it. . . .

I wish I could understand it. Sex is wonderful, but I got too caught up in it. I know that sounds like a cop-out, but it all felt so good while I was doing it. I wasn't thinking straight. I know better. I know all about HIV and how it's transmitted. I've seen a lot of people in late stages of AIDS. I know better, and I don't want that [AIDS] to happen to me. I just got out of control. I always try to practice safer sex, and I haven't had unsafe sex since. I hope it won't happen again. But who knows? It might if I don't watch out, but I am always prepared. I have my condom and lube out where it's easy to get to. I know this sounds stupid, but sometimes during sex I become real obsessed.

Experiences with Death and People Living with AIDS

Jerry has been deeply affected by death and loss due to the epidemic's ravages in the gay community. He has lost several acquaintances, but the most devastating loss for him was the death of his ex-lover Jack. Unlike Roger in the previous chapter, Jerry has no sense or thoughts that he will inevitably become infected. In fact, at one point he stated that he will never understand what it is like to be HIV positive and later insisted, with much elation and bravado, that he will survive the epidemic.

God, I wish it [AIDS] would go away. If I were still religious, I would pray every night to make it go away. I've lost so many acquaintances. One minute they're laughing and partying, and the next minute they're in a gurney hooked up to an IV or something. I go to a party and you hear about so-and-so being sick or so-and-so dying or so-and-so being in mourning.

I don't get depressed about it. I just go on and push forward. I try to keep my sense of humor and laugh. That's a very good thing about being gay. It's as if we've got some kind of mission not to let AIDS get us down, to survive and to laugh in its face. I want to survive, and I want to keep laughing. I'm going to survive this epidemic come hell or high water.

I did get a little depressed after Jack died. He was such a sweet man. I got through it. I feel so lucky to have known such a wonderful and kind man. I even remember our fights and how stupid and downright silly they all were, but I don't regret leaving him. We made better friends than lovers. I helped his family make a panel for the AIDS quilt and that helped me—and I think his family too—a lot. I have his memories and that's how I keep him alive. Always with me.

I still have friends who are HIV positive, but I have to admit, I am hesitant about making a really close gay friendship because I can't be sure they won't die on me. I know that sounds tacky, but I don't want to get too close to someone else and then have to say goodbye. It's never easy.

I'll never understand what it is like to be HIV positive. I can only guess that it is horrible to realize that your life will probably be cut short. I admire my HIV-positive friends who still enjoy life. [In that] we have something in common. We refuse to let this epidemic ruin us, and we make the most of our situations.

Want to hear something funny and personal? [*I nod, as if nothing else he had told me was personal*] When AIDS gets me down, I just keep singing that old Gloria Gaynor disco song from the seventies. You remember that one, don't you? [*He begins to sing*] "I will survive. As long as I know how to love, I know I'll stay alive. I've got all my life to live. I've got so much love to give. I will survive." God, I love that song. You remember that one. Don't you?

I do remember that song, and as his second and last interview came to a close, Jerry and I sat for what seemed to be no less than a minute from eternity, intensely concentrating in an endeavor to recall each and every melodic word while belting way off key in voices less like Gloria Gaynor's and more like Tom Arnold's. Together we laughed in the wake of an epidemic, optimistic that our voices would somehow constrain the virus and that Gloria Gaynor's prophecy, fomented in a swarm of disco madness, would come true.

8

Theorizing Sexual Pleasure: Fuzzy, Evolutionary, and Cultural

All around us things change their identities. The atoms that make up the universe swirl and collide and keep swirling and colliding. Everything is in flux. Everything flows. The universe unfolds as a river runs. The cosmological fluid seems to obey Einstein's laws of general relativity in the large and seems to obey the laws of quantum mechanics in the small and obeys we do not know what in between. . . . We can put black and white labels on things. But the labels will pass from accurate to inaccurate as the things change.

—Bart Kosko, *Fuzzy Thinking* (1993)

The essence of romance is uncertainty.

—Oscar Wilde, quoted in Diane Ackerman, *A Natural History of Love* (1994)

Consensual sex is pleasurable for most people, and pleasure, like pain, is a subjective sensation. Individuals crave pleasure, but where they find it at any given moment depends upon, at least in part, their own personal and subjective tastes (Ackerman 1994). Like all human beings, the gay men who have shared their stories in this book hunger for some degree of sexual pleasure, but the locations they choose and methods they utilize vary, with no apparent underlying pattern. It is evident that all of them enjoy sex, and yet, one man longs for novel sex with someone other than his lover, one likes pleasing his partner by way of an "electrical" spiritual connection, one craves pornographic fantasy, one is pleasure-curious, and one relishes the fetishistic appeal of leather. Some of them like being penetrated anally, some prefer to penetrate, and some like both. Some enjoy oral sex, some play with sex toys, and some find pleasure in lengthy foreplay.

Not only does the pursuit and meaning of pleasure apparently vary across individuals; it is also fluid through time and space for any given person. For most of these men, learning to explore a spectrum of new sexual play during the "good old days" of the 1970s altered to varying degrees their individually desired sexual acts and potential partners. By way of experimentation, each man acquired a personalized smorgasbord of new sexual pleasures, such as the use of leather, anal penetration, kissing, and other behaviors preferred in differing contexts. For some, these preferences continued to change after the advent of AIDS awareness. Bob, for example, acquired an appetite for oral sex, leaving anal sex behind as a pleasure of the past. For Phil in chapter 4, just the fact of growing older, in and of itself, influenced his lustful preferences. As the years advanced, he went from wanting older men to being attracted to younger ones.

It is this variability both within and between individuals that, on the surface, creates the appearance of the lack of a pattern to this group of men's unsafer sexual encounters. There is nothing to indicate or reassure us that instances of unsafer sex occur in any kind of orderly, predictable fashion. Rather the how, when, where, and why such episodes of unsafer sex take place remains maddeningly fuzzy.

Beneath this confusing blur of behavior, however, may be found some general salient unsafer sex commonalities. Consider, for example, that in this group of men condoms were readily accessible to all but one man. All did not discuss safer sex up-front before embarking upon their heated sexual encounter, and the unsafer sex was unanimously spontaneous. Additionally, they were all in a state of heightened arousal, and each found the unsafer event more pleasurable; but, after the fact, they expressed grievous remorse for having put themselves in such a risky situation.

Many of these comprehensive descriptive themes have been presented in other studies of gay male sexual behaviors (see chapter 1), but are of limited use in their application to individuals since they are actually mere abstractions from the particularized context of specific and authentic sexual encounters. As such, they are more like course grains of generalization, the result of methodologies that ignore the more finely sifted realities of fuzzy variation. Moreover, these thematic connections and their relative importance can only be located within each man's own experience as he slides through an ever-changing continuum of time and space leading from less risky to more risky sex.

Put another way, gay men's sexual stories (like anyone else's) really present a picture of the all-encompassing variations of life, which is the muddled world of decision-making and sexual experience as rooted in subjective pleasure in whatever form it may manifest at any given point in time. Pleasure, then, is an aesthetic experience formed by each individual's own sexual life pathway—one's culture, relations, situations, and experiences—but it is also, not inconsequentially, an evolved biological high for which the human animal yearns.

Evolution and Pleasure

There has been much ado among a small group of evolutionary biologists and anthropologists intrigued by the role of sex in human evolution. And for good reason. Without sex, *Homo sapiens sapiens* (human beings) would not be able to reproduce themselves, thereby passing on their DNA legacy—quite possibly in combination with new and novel mutations—to the next generation. The paradigm under which researchers and students of evolution operate is a theory described by Charles Darwin in 1859 when he wrote *On the Origin of Species by Natural Selection*. His theory, though simple in its outlines, marked an immense leap forward in our understanding of how we as human beings have come to be and, in some cases, why we do what we do.

Darwin's theory rests upon the process of natural selection, best described using three basic postulates: (1) the ability of a population to grow is infinite, but the capacity of the environment to hold a population is finite; (2) individuals vary in their ability to survive and reproduce (some individuals are more adapted to their *current* environment than are others); and (3) this variation is heritable.

It is primarily the second of these postulates that lead "adaptationists" to propose that the purpose of sex is for reproduction, for passing on an individual's genes to the next generation (Cronin 1991; Dawkins 1989; Ridley 1993). Heterosexual behaviors fit neatly under this proposition, but it is obviously impossible for two men to reproduce in the "old-fashioned" sense (i.e., without surrogate mothers and artificial insemination).

Because of this, homosexuality has complicated evolutionary theories of sex. The impossibility of two men reproducing and passing on their DNA, along with the existence of many other nonreproductive human sexual behaviors—even heterosexual sex can be nonreproductive—has prompted Abramson and Pinkerton (1995) to suggest that the ultimate evolutionary function of sex may be for reproduction in order to propagate genes but that "the proximal motivation for engaging in sex is usually the pursuit of pleasure rather than a conscious desire to procreate. . . . The explanatory power of pleasure—as a conceptual framework for analyzing human sexual behavior—far exceeds that of reproduction. . . . The biology of pleasure seems relatively more obscure than the sociology of pleasure" (10–11).

Thus there may be an evolved drive for sexual pleasure, which provides a contributive and explanatory area for research on the variety of pleasurable human sexual behaviors that exist throughout the world (regardless if the sexual encounters are reproductive or not).

Unfortunately, as Abramson and Pinkerton allude to above, little is understood about the physiological basis of sexual pleasure and its drive. Perhaps it is disturbing for humans to think that something as personal as sexual desires (often associated with love) could partially stem from a biological predisposition to seek out pleasure. Likewise, especially in cultures based on a Judeo-Christian ethos, the biblical focus upon reproduction over pleasure may color theoretical approaches to sex.

Some researchers dismiss biological explanations of human sexuality because they worry that such interpretations will prompt biomedicine to label individuals with "unacceptable" urges as pathological or that individuals will use their biology as an excuse for potentially destructive behaviors (Davies et al. 1993; Odets 1995); or, worse, that biological explanations will provide ammunition to eugenicist movements that may want to "clean" the gene pool of genes socioculturally defined as deleterious (see Drlica 1994).

These are valid concerns and I will touch upon them shortly as I review what little is currently known about the human neurophysiological response to sexual arousal. For now, I will simply emphasize that, in the midst of a virulent sexually transmitted disease pandemic, the cost of ignoring potential biological factors pertaining to sexual behaviors may have an even greater deleterious impact.

What's more, contrary to popular belief, a biological predisposition does not equal an outcome. There is more to the equation. Biology is not deterministic as it also interacts with environment and culture to create the complexity of a human being (Abramson and Pinkerton 1995). It is not nature (biology) versus nurture (environment/culture/society), but nature *and* nurture. The relationship between nature and nurture is interactive—and fuzzy. The degree of influence for both nature and nurture probably depends upon the phenomenon in question. However, to ignore biology, or any other component of human behavior for that matter, is to be like one of the lost characters of *The Wizard of Oz*, each of them searching for an important piece necessary to make them into what they wish to become, only to realize in the end that what they needed was with them the entire time. "Don't pay any attention to the man behind the curtain," said the Wizard (who was the man behind the curtain).

Physical Responses to Sexual Pleasure and Rationality: Caught in the Moment

As a result of the dearth of information available about the biological drive for and the physiological impact of sexual pleasure, I must here venture into a somewhat speculative discussion, but I will draw upon a few intriguing studies in biology, neurobiology, and human evolution. Needless to say, much more research in this area is sorely needed.

As I have already emphasized, pleasure reinforces sexual behaviors that are important for reproduction whether or not the intent of the act is for reproduction every time. Thus sexual pleasure, in and of itself, is neither good nor bad. It is a natural response, but the consequences of pleasure will vary within any given environment, culture, society, or for a given individual. The atavistic thirst for sexual pleasure probably evolved in a different world and environment than exists today. It was a prehistoric world in which small groups of humans made their living as hunters and gatherers on an African plain and in which many modern microbes, including sexually transmitted ones, did not exist in large numbers. In prehistory, a drive for sexual pleasure would not have contributed to a deadly epidemic, but instead would have increased human reproduction and would have conceivably contributed to the formation of social bonds and group alliances (Bailey and Aunger 1995; Neese and Williams 1994).

Today, however, we do not live in the same environment as did our hunting and gathering ancestors. There are larger human populations, sometimes packed into large urban centers. As human populations grew more dense, human microbes, including sexually transmitted ones, were provided with an ample environment of human hosts in which to flourish (Ewald 1994; Garrett 1994; Lappé 1995). As Richard Preston (1994) so graphically puts it in his book *The Hot Zone*, "The extreme amplification of the human race, which has occurred only in the past hundred years or so, has suddenly produced a very large quantity of meat, which is sitting everywhere in the biosphere and may not be able to defend itself against a life form [microbes] that might want to consume it" (287).

The human need for sex and its carnal rewards may be problematic in this novel modern environment burdened by its population of over five billion *Homo sapien sapiens* and in which sexually transmitted organisms thrive, often beyond our immediate detection. Our bodies are designed for pleasure, not for tracking diseases (Bailey and Aunger 1995; Neese and Williams 1994).

Our propensity to seek out sexual pleasure is not the only evolved craving which has contributed, in some cases, to poor health outcomes. For example, hunters and gatherers went to great lengths to find sugar, salt, and fat, which were in short supply or were difficult to procure. Yet all of these substances are important to the human diet. Therefore, a drive to want more, to go out and secure these substances—spending much time and energy while doing so—would be adaptive in our ancestors' environments. Now, however, these substances are plentiful in some parts of the world, particularly in the industrialized nations. The environment has changed, but we still have a drive to crave more, a drive that can lead to poor health outcomes including obesity, cavities, hypertension, clogged arteries, and diabetes (see Neese and Williams 1994). Just as with human hankerings for sugar, salt, and fat, within our current environment—

overcrowded and infectious—our drive for sexual pleasure can reek unhealthy havoc.

Nonetheless, our bodies have evolved psychobiological responses to sexual experience and encounters in which hormones and enzymes, in response to arousal, in a sense rush to tell us: "Go for it. This feels good." By way of evolution, our bodies are well designed for receiving and giving sexual pleasure. Once an individual anticipates (desires) and then becomes enveloped in a pleasurable sexual experience, the senses (vision, smell, hearing, taste, and touch) are stimulated.

As demonstrated by the gay men's sexual experiences described in previous chapters, these types of sensual stimuli are multitudinous but can be classified under five domains. All five domains are part of the acting out of individual fantasies leading to sexual arousal as neurons fire and one's body chemistry transforms.

The first of these domains, environmental stimulation, can contribute to pleasure whether it be pornography displayed in the sensorial background, leather decor, a particular meeting place with sexually stimulating music and lighting, or as one group of researchers has suggested, even the wallpaper pattern where the encounter occurs (Davies et al. 1993).

Sexual accessories like leather gloves, whips, dildos, and other sex toys endow both partners with a chest of tools to please each other, greatening the pleasurable impact of the human sexual bond.

Blending with the environment and sexual paraphernalia, the sexual partner's physical characteristics add to the experience. Having one's eyes behold the body type or penis shape and size that one desires as well as a particular partner's height, hand size, hair color, eye color, or something as subtle as the shape of a chin, all heighten sexual arousal.

But the sexual partner is more than just physical characteristics. He has experience, sexual abilities, and puts on a sexual performance, which, depending upon the desires of each member of the sexual union, can stir passion into the moment. With differing partners, the sex may be more or less "wild," slow and romantic, electric, or "hot."

As the sexual conversation heightens, interactive sensory stimulation—such as smelling perfumes, body sweat, leather, and incense, or audio bombardment from the sounds of mild spanking, groaning, and animal-like growls, all accompanied by the taste of a penis, an anus, or another man's lips, the touch or feel of skin and penetration—lead one closer to orgasm. Milder and stronger mind-altering substances such as alcohol, marijuana, or poppers may provide backup to the enhanced blend of neural stimulation.

It is no scientific secret that sensory stimulation can excite pleasure centers in our brain, and in sexual encounters, sensory stimulation begins when two partners first lock eyes (Ackerman 1994; LeVay 1994; Restak 1994; Schmidt 1983). From the moment of first contact, the sexual encounter is a form of communication (Daniel and Parker 1993; Davies et al. 1993), and this communication involves all five senses, producing a brilliant fireworks display of neuronal activity (LeVay 1994; Restak 1994). When an "attractive" sexual partner is first sighted, a person feels a rush of excitement, bordering on euphoria, brought on by a flood of phenylethylamine (PEA), an amphetamine-like substance that humans appear to crave (Liebowitz 1983). And so sexual arousal begins.

Other chemical changes also occur during arousal. Research on drugs for the treatment of sexual "dysfunctions" such as impotence and lack of sexual desire have provided clues to the potential role of chemical substances in sexual arousal. Researchers have tested a variety of drugs that alter the level of neurotransmitters, the chemical messengers of the brain, and these studies have rendered some interesting results (Rosen and Ashton 1992).

One of the more studied messengers, at least in regard to sexual arousal and desire, is dopamine. Dopamine has received more attention because the depletion of dopamine in one area of the brain has been implicated as a possible factor in the tremors and rigidity of limbs associated with Parkinson's disease and, further, when at abnormally high levels in the brain, dopamine may play a role in schizophrenia (Restak 1994; Schneider and Tarshis 1986). However, the possible prosexual effects of drugs that increase levels of dopamine in the brain include increased sexual desire and arousal, improved nocturnal erections, and an increase in the number of erections (Rosen and Ashton 1992).

Male sexual drive can also be decreased and increased by varying levels of the adrenal sex hormone, testosterone. Once aroused, the brain signals the adrenal gland to release sex hormones which then feed back to the brain, stimulating sexual behavior (Schneider and Tarshis 1986). John Money (1961) used adrenal sex hormones to treat men with underactive testes. As a result of the hormones, the men experienced an increase in sexual activity, and this activity lapsed when the therapy was discontinued.

Moreover, during a man's orgasm, massive amounts of the hormone oxytocin are released, perhaps under the control of the endorphin system, flooding him with body-twitching pleasure. There is an increase in his heart rate, blood pressure, muscle tension, and a rosy sexual flush rises over his chest, thighs, arms, shoulders, neck, and face, giving the appearance of a rash (Masters and Johnson 1966).

Part of a man's sexual response may also be linked to a tiny section of the brain, the hypothalamus, representing less than 1 percent of total brain volume and found nestled between the limbic area and the cerebral cortex. The limbic area of the brain is the oldest part of the human brain and is the processing plant for human emotions. The cerebral cortex, on the other hand, is where logic and higher-level thought take place. The hypothalamus, weighing in at around four grams, forms a critical link between the two and regulates some of the most fundamental aspects of physical survival, including hormone levels, water balance, temperature, appetite, and sexual activity (LeVay 1994; Restak 1994).

The hypothalamus is essential to sex, and this is the primary area of the brain where activity involving sex hormones takes place. In the 1960s, West German men whose sexual behaviors were deemed pathological had their hypothalamic nuclei destroyed. Afterward, they not only lost their ability to perform sexually, but their sexual *desires*, *fantasies*, and *drives* were also reduced (LeVay 1994). According to Simon LeVay (1994), the hypothalamus not only receives sensory information from the cortex about our environment and our desires; it also influences the cortex, sending back signals that influence sexual ideation and complex sexual behaviors.

In addition to the hypothalamus, Richard Cytowic (1993) has suggested, based upon his work with people who have the condition known as synesthesia, that when activity in the limbic (emotional) area of the brain is increased, there is a reduction in the activity of the cortex (thought) area, and vice versa. He writes: "The role of the cortex is to analyze the external world and contain our model of reality. It is the limbic brain [emotion], however, that decides questions of salience and relevance and so determines how we act on the information we have" (159).

Be it the hypothalamus, the limbic brain, sex hormones, endorphins, and/or neurotransmitters, perhaps one or more of these perspectives about how the human brain functions and the chemical bases of sex can provide an explanation for the results of an experiment performed on a group of college age women. The women were given a math test. As they crunched away at the numbers, these women certainly required the use of their cerebral cortexes in order to think in the logical realm of mathematics. Next they were shown erotic videos to promote sexual arousal. Afterward, they took the test again and the second time around their scores were notably reduced (Lyon 1993). This could be interpreted to mean that, following arousal, the women's ability to perform mathematical logic, upon which risk calculation is based, was somewhat impaired. Put another way, their ability to think logically was somewhat reduced, but not totally eliminated, after sexual arousal.

Coming back to the men in this book, it is quite possible that their ability to think logically is inversely related to the degree of sexual pleasure experienced. The more pleasure, the less rationality, and most sexual encounters probably fall somewhere in the middle of the spectrum (i.e., partly logical and partly pleasurable). Thus in some situations in which arousal is heightened to a greater degree, they "lose control." In other cases like that of Alexander in chapter 5, he may make a decision to forgo a condom because it is too tight for his partner, inhibiting the sexual "electricity." He may mingle logic and pleasure.

To be sure, some sexual encounters are more or less exhilarating, thrilling, and spine-tingling, and a man's body and his brain potentially respond accordingly. He is stimulated to some degree from beginning to end, and as some of the men in this study describe their unsafer experiences, if he is highly stimulated he may become "caught in the moment" or "wild," becoming lost in a rush of "excitement" culminating in orgasm. During sexual arousal, it is not that he is "turned on" or "not turned on." Some sexual encounters may arouse him more than others, and hence he may be more or less "turned on."

Notwithstanding this fuzzy response, most of the men who reported unprotected sex did not place their risk of HIV infection in the forefront of their thoughts while engaged in the act. It is true that some, but not all, did attempt to reduce their risk by pulling out before ejaculation, but I am suggesting here the possibility of a reduction in the ability to think logically or rationally, not a complete blackout of cognitive function. Tossing out Aristotelian logic, we may conceive that the aroused male is both logical and illogical, rational and irrational, at the same time.

Which brings me to another issue in sex and behavioral research about risky behaviors for HIV infection. Researchers and community activists often debate whether unsafer sex is rational or irrational, but the debate, as so often is the case, is based upon black and white categorizations: sex is rational or it is irrational—with no middle ground.

Davies et al. (1993) argue that having unsafer sex "is not necessarily due to a failure of rationality, but to the logic of the sexual conversation dominating over the logic of safety. . . . This is not necessarily irrational." Still and all, reality is probably fuzzier than this analysis permits. One form of rationality feasibly does not replace another. Instead, some sex is potentially more or less rational than other sex, and unsafer sex is less rational than safer sex. Instead of one type of logic replacing another or irrationality taking charge of a man's actions, it may be that the logic of safety is simply reduced by the sexual conversation and the five sexual domains leading to arousal that I outlined above. Rationality and irrationality mingle into a fuzzy erotic cocktail.

However, to suggest a reduction in logic, as I am doing here, is not the same as labeling individuals as "deficient," "pathological," "incapable," or viewing them as "the other" (Davies et al. 1993; Odets 1995). I am labeling these men as human, not as the other, by putting forth that gay men are subject to the same evolutionary desires and psychobiological sexual responses that are in varying degrees part of the makeup of human males (and females, one can presume) regardless of sexuality. And in any case, the sexually aroused man's logic may be *somewhat* deficient in the sexual moment, but he is not incapable of practicing safer sex most of the time. He is not a pathological anomaly.

Nor am I suggesting that biology provides a male excuse for unsafer sex (Levine and Siegel 1992). To the contrary, biology is only one piece of the sexual puzzle. We are not total slaves to physical drives. As Abramson and Pinkerton point out, despite this evolved drive, "People are largely free to choose when, how, and with whom they have sex" (1995:10). This free choice is best exemplified by the story of Bob, the only man here who said that he had not had anal sex without a condom in the recent past. When Bob is engrossed in a sexual encounter and feels that unsafer sex could occur, he turns on a little voice in his head and stops regardless of what the other partner wants. He has learned and adopted a skill to prevent his getting "caught in the moment," to help him control his drives, and to modify his behaviors.

Unlike some other animals, humans are not "controlled" by basic drives. We have a cortex and we have culture. Both play a role, along with biology, in the expression of our drives for sexual pleasure (Abramson and Pinkerton 1995; Tuzin 1995). We just have to use these resources to our advantage.

Interaction: Nature and Nurture

It is important to note that I have here been talking about pleasure derived from behaviors, not about identity. After all, it is well known by anthropologists who look at sexual behaviors cross-culturally that male-male and female-female sex may occur in the absence of a gay identity (Carrier 1977, 1980; Greenberg 1988; Herdt 1984, 1987); and conversely, though less studied, male-female sex can presumably take place in the absence of a heterosexual identity (Browning 1994).

Nevertheless, during my biological discussion of unsafer sexual behaviors and pleasure, critics of functional explanations, particularly social constructionists, are surely muttering with polite furor, "Well, what about culture?" Of course, culture and human experience also play a role. It would be naive and simple—just as it is to ignore biology—to think otherwise. As I have said before (but which bears repeating lest I be misunderstood), biology and culture are not opposites but instead are interactive (Kosko 1993; Tuzin 1995). It is not nature versus nurture but rather the excluded middle of nature and nurture that contributes to human sexual behaviors and sexuality—but the relationship between the two may vary depending upon the phenomenon under study.

In regard to the phenomenon at hand, unsafer sex and pleasure, there is probably a human biological drive to seek pleasure, while culture and life experience also play a role by providing meaning to the sexual encounter for the individual as well as by providing ways of expressing and ways of constraining sexual behaviors (Abramson and Pinkerton 1995; Edgerton 1992; Greenberg 1995; Meyer-Bahlberg 1995; Udry 1988; Weinrich et al. 1993). Put simply, culture allows for and provides defined pleasurable experiences.

Jerry, for example, in chapter 7 finds pleasure in leather and domination. There could be at least two cultural explanations for his tastes. First, gay culture is a more sex-positive culture that allows for a great deal of sexual expression without too much inhibition. Therefore, Jerry's delectation in mild spanking and in using leather stimulants are acceptable and allowed in gay culture, not prohibited, taboo, or something about which to feel guilty. Second, gay culture provides settings for experiencing sexual rewards from a variety of pleasurable sources. Thus Jerry's hangout, the Spike, a gay man's Levi's/leather bar, provides an appropriate place to meet other men adorned in leather, the ultimate source of Jerry's pleasure.

Culture may also constrict biological drives to a degree. For example, anthropologist Robert Edgerton (1992) proposes that there is a basic human drive for novelty—the need to escape boredom—which culture attempts to constrain. This drive can lead to "socially disruptive, deviant behavior as people violate what they experience as stifling cultural constraints" (73). The need to escape boredom, however, may be little more than the need for pleasure, at least as far as sexual pleasure goes, as sexual pleasure can be found in novelty. As Diane Ackerman writes, "Sometimes our senses wantonly crave novelty, for no other reason than that it feels good" (1994:165).

Johnny, in chapter 2, sought out novel sexual partners and found them to be most pleasurable. As he put it, "Sometimes I just want to try something new, explore a new body, something novel. Don't misunderstand me. I love Ralph [his lover] more than I have ever loved anyone. We do a lot of different things together sexually, but it's not the same as touching an unknown, unexplored body."

However, the *ideal* American cultural norm of monogamy places restrictions on his drive even if there are occasional transgressions. In gay culture, there is a tension between norms of sexual liberation and the norms of monogamy which are taught to gay men during their youth. One set of norms allows total expression of the drive for pleasure while the other attempts to constrain it, and it is this tension which lies behind Johnny's description of his "monogamous" relationship as a "sacrifice," a sacrifice of pleasure.

Johnny is not alone in his management of opposing cultural norms. As told in chapter 4, Phil goes on sexual binges after extended periods of abstinence by basking in the sexual ambiance permissible to him as a gay man; but he also lives within a non-gay, Judeo-Christian-based culture in which such expressions are judged and prohibited (Foucault 1978), which leads him to long bouts of abstinence, guilt, and fear. Phil rides binge-and-purge cycles trying desperately to control physically gratifying behaviors that are culturally "unacceptable" but, at the same time, are culturally available.

For other gay men such prohibition may also have an opposite impact. Making a behavior forbidden sometimes increases the pleasure associated with the naughtiness or danger of the act, as it did for Roger with his curiosity about unprotected sex, the prohibited behavior that he had never experienced (Browning 1994; Vance 1984). The association between prohibition, danger, and pleasure may also partially account for why all the men here described unsafer anal sex without a condom as being more enjoyable. Above and beyond the apparent physical reduction in pleasure that occurs when a latex barrier covers the highly sensitive skin of the penis during intercourse, breaking the safer sex taboo and its associated risk may heighten the pleasurable meaning of the experience.

Culture, then, provides the setting for sexual encounters, impacts the meaning of specific acts, and provides sexual constraints upon (but also allows for) sexual expression. These cultural influences increase and decrease pleasure. This does not deny but instead reinforces the argument that there is an interaction between culture and the biological drive or motivation to search out sexual pleasure. Culture may impact what we find to be pleasurable and its expression, but our physiological response and drive lead us to seek out that pleasure.

Health Education, Relapse, and Abstinence

As a part of American middle-class culture, health education in the United States generally attempts to change cultural norms and individual behaviors in order to provide constraints on evolutionary behaviors, encouraging us to adapt to our modern environment. Health education as a profession struggles to regulate our evolutionary drives for pleasure through sex, food, drugs (including tobacco), and alcohol as well as a myriad of thrill-seeking behaviors which may put us at risk for harm. This task requires a zealous commitment, and it has the potential for helping individuals adapt to a changing environment that includes HIV.

Nonetheless, some researchers, including myself, have criticized health education approaches on the basis of their Judeo-Christian values: "Two millennia of Christian thought have deeply ingrained in the Western mind a belief in the subservience of the body to will and have led to the belief that the body's demands—lust, thirst, pleasure, etc.—are undesirable, evil and subhuman drives" (Davies et al. 1993:49; also see Turner 1994).

Clearly the behaviors targeted by health educators (gluttony, sexual license, drunkenness, and so-called other "sins") are also targets of most Judeo-Christian-based religions. Still and all, just because a value system is based upon Judeo-Christian thought does not mean that it is a complete and total fallacy or inherently bad. Religion, as part of a culture, can provide adaptive benefits by regulating our relationship with our environment (Harris 1979), and as is the case with unsafer sex and HIV infection, maintaining some degree of control may indeed prevent dire consequences.

The real issue, however, is not religious attempts to control biological urges, but instead has to do with the tendency of Judeo-Christian-based culture (as well as the tendency of its critics) to see the world in stark black-and-white terms. As I suggested in the introduction, this problem clearly predates Christianity. It is not Judeo-Christian thought per se which may be detrimental to (for example) health education but rather the application of Aristotle's law of the excluded middle and the law of noncontradiction to a fuzzy world in which individuals make fuzzy decisions about the performance of fuzzy behaviors, including sexual ones.

It is true that in their mandate to promote health and to prevent new HIV infections, health educators might use a variety of methods and theories (Levinton 1989), but for the most part they share a common understanding of the nature of reality. This nature of reality is grounded in the use of binary categories and all-or-nothing approaches. Since the beginning of the epidemic, the debate surrounding sex and HIV prevention has been polarized (Valdiserri 1989). Sten Vermund in an editorial in the *American Journal of Public Health* aptly describes this "destructive" debate. He writes: "Many good persons of good will urge risk elimination through mutual monogamy (assuming an HIV-seronegative, non-drug-using partner) or celibacy, while others advocate risk reduction through more selective choice in sexual relations and the use of barriers" (1995:1488).

These two poles of the public health debate represent all-or-nothing, binary categories. The first position of risk elimination represents the "nothing." To promote condoms, the abstinence argument goes, will encourage sex outside of marriage. Therefore, to protect themselves, people had better get hitched or just be celibate.

Superficially, the alternative position of risk reduction appears to be somewhat fuzzy, but in its implementation it is often the "all" approach. In past health education seminars that I have given, designed, or attended, an HIV risk continuum (from most safe to least safe) is often presented to program participants; but as soon as the program begins, the conversation splits the continuum into two categories. Suddenly a continuum becomes safer and unsafe—with safer being anal sex and/or oral sex with a condom while unsafe is any penetration without a condom. Risk reduction in this circumstance is here narrowed to mean *always* using a condom for any and every type of penetration.

Thus the debate described by Sten Vermund actually boils down to a choice between condoms for all forms of penetration every time (*or* all) versus monogamy/celibacy (*or* nothing). Both of these positions defy the continuum of risk, but gay men, at least in their behaviors, do not follow either. All the men in this book practice oral sex without a condom as a risk-reduction strategy. For Bob, it gives him the pleasure of penetration without the higher degree of risk associated with anal sex without a condom. He has reduced his risk, but according to some HIV prevention programs he has not. In the view of these programs, he is absolutely still at risk.

In regard to oral sex, the behavior of gay men and the application of risk reduction by some health educators (as I have described it) represent two different perceptions of risk. Levine and Siegel (1992) make a distinction between the public health construction of risk versus the "folk" construction of risk. They point out that in the folk construction of risk, pre-ejaculatory fluids (pre-cum) and the urethral opening are not suitable routes for transmission because saliva and gastric acids neutralize the virus and that there is documented evidence for such beliefs. The folk construction was evident in most of my interviews with gay men. Maintaining an awareness of the condition of their teeth and gums in relation to oral sex was considered by most of those interviewed to be adequate risk reduction, as was pulling out before ejaculation during anal intercourse.

But there is an ambiguous line between the public health model of risk and the folk model of risk as incorporated into the behaviors of many gay men. Gay men do not buy the "all" approach of health education, which though called "risk reduction" is actually risk elimination (see Donovan et al. 1995). Gay men for the most part, though, have incorporated safer sex information into their sexual repertoire and have reduced, if not eliminated altogether, their risk of infection; but some health educators are still not pleased.

At one Los Angeles community-based organization, I was called "a murderer" by one health educator for even suggesting that oral sex should be taught as a risk-reduction strategy. In 1993, at this same agency, I observed focus groups featuring an erotic safer sex video from Great Britain. The focus groups consisted of AIDS service providers and health educators. Many of the group's participants generally liked the film but thought that it was too lenient in its description of oral sex without a condom. The film noted that there may be some risk, but that it was probably lower than the risk associated with anal sex without a condom; yet many health educators in the room sat with their arms crossed, frowning at the two actors on the screen—one giving fellatio without a condom to the other. It had to be all or nothing.

Dissenters from this extreme position are becoming more vocal, however, and even the State of California has funded at least one program that I know of which targets homeless teens and explicitly teaches oral sex as a risk-reduction strategy. Other programs are beginning to adopt this perspective as well, including the above-noted community-based organization.

I would be amiss not to point out that the elimination approach is not a universal one. Health educators and researchers from Great Britain, parts of Europe, and Australia, many of them cited throughout this book, have already taken up a risk-reduction approach. In other countries, oral sex is considered and often taught as an acceptable risk-reduction strategy. Government-funded posters portraying two men entwined in oral sex and inscribed with safer sex messages were praised early on (for example, in Germany).

Still, risk reduction is more than teaching oral sex as a less risky activity and needs to address the main behavior of concern for the men in this book: occasional unprotected anal sex. To do so requires one to place the infrequent unsafer sex event in the context of a life-long sexual history. In this history, given my evolutionary argument, many (but not all) gay men may have a sporadic unsafer sex experience when in a heightened state of arousal. Instead of slapping on all-or-nothing labels such as "relapser" or "lapser," which only truly make sense for that one specific experience, safer sex should be viewed as a process, one in which risk is reduced but probably not always eliminated. Thus a man who used to have unsafer sex all the time, but has since reduced the frequency of unprotected anal sex to a rare event, is *not* a lapser or a relapser. He is a man who has reduced his risk.

To sum up thus far before moving to a discussion about specific interventions: by having reduced their frequency of unsafer sex experiences since the 1970s, the gay men in this book have indeed succeeded in reducing their risk. They practice safer sex most of the time as they attempt to adhere to the new social norm of safer sex (Hospers and Kok 1995). But the norm also has a downside. The problem is that social norms are attempting to restrict a basic drive, a drive for sexual pleasure. Given this, there may always be occasional degrees of transgression (slips) from the norm, with the frequency and types of slips varying among individuals. Though presented with the best of intentions, the black-and-white, all-or-nothing approach of some health educators—which recognizes only success (safer sex all the time) or failure (relapse/lapse)—is founded upon ideal philosophies and transient definitions, not upon the ongoing, living contradictions of the real world.

One can abandon these labels, however, and still develop effective interventions. One can also propose a biological predisposition or component to any behavior that has health consequences without surrendering to, "well it's natural so there's nothing you can do." Unsafer sex has an evolved biological component, but it is not the only determining factor. Human beings have a degree of free will, social organization, and culture. As I will demonstrate in the next chapter, these additional factors can help us to reach an optimal, if not perfect, adaptation to a dangerous environment harboring a deadly sexually transmitted disease or they can lead us, individually and collectively, down the path to a slow but steady demise.

9 Adapting to HIV: Intervention Strategies

> We shape the diseases that afflict us as much as they have shaped us. Taking responsibility for modern diseases such as AIDS, TB, and Lyme disease requires that we once again step back and recognize the role we have played in their emergence. While it may not be possible to turn back the clock, we can nonetheless restore the balanced relationships that kept these diseases in check over the millennia. This means incorporating evolutionary strategies into their control.
>
> —Marc Lappé, *Break Out* (1995)

> You must always remember to go home without it [sex]. Those are the times that you have to remember that other times you will have it and it doesn't matter if sometimes you don't have it and have to go home without it, go home alone without it, go home alone without it, go home without it.
>
> —Tennessee Williams, "Hard Candy" (1954)

It has been said over and over again that in the absence of a vaccine, health education and prevention are our only hope to stop (perhaps slow is more appropriate) the AIDS epidemic. Slowing the epidemic requires that individuals and groups adapt to a new infectious world. In this chapter, I will suggest approaches to help gay men adapt to HIV, but before doing so, there are four caveats I urge you to keep in mind.

First, I am making these recommendations only for interventions targeting gay men who have already adopted safer sex but continue to have occasional unsafer sex (those men who have been labeled "relapsers" or "lapsers"). I am not advocating the same approach for other groups as there is not a one-shot method that will work for everyone (Valdiserri 1989).

Second, by presenting possible interventions, I am advocating maintenance of safer sex practices most of the time, recognizing that there are no perfect human beings of any race, gender, cultural group, or sexuality. Sometimes things do not go as planned or as we would like them to proceed, and there is a degree of unpredictability, as well as a degree of predictability, in many situations or events. My intervention suggestions are offered solely to provide potential ways in which the number of unsafer sex events within an individual's lifetime can be kept at a minimal level (i.e., rare within the context of the individual's sexual life).

Third, I will be attributing a degree of personal responsibility to the individual to manage his behavior. I am certain that the mere suggestion of this will lead some of my colleagues to scoff and accuse me of "blaming the victim" (Ryan 1971), so I had best explain my perspective. It is not that an individual is a victim or not a victim, or that a person is responsible or not responsible. Both the notion of blaming the victim and the idea of personal responsibility offer examples of extreme linguistic categories in popular American political debate. In a fuzzy reality, an individual can be a victim to a degree and still play a role in his or her own victimization (i.e., a responsible victim). Besides, attributing a degree of responsibility is *not* the same as blaming someone for their behavior, but instead provides a way to empower them so that they can maintain a degree of control over their situation, their relations, their role in sexual communication, and their own body by developing individualized approaches to self-management. As health psychologist Albert Bandura writes, "Translating health knowledge into effective self-protection action against AIDS infection requires social skills and a sense of personal power to exercise control over sexual situations" (1989:129).

Finally, it should be glaringly apparent that in this book I have presented only one participant's side in the sexual conversation. By doing so, I may be falling into what some researchers have labeled as "the individualistic fallacy," the attempt to understand sexual behavior by looking at one person alone (Davies et al. 1993). Obviously, it takes more than one person to have sex, but—it only takes *one* person to stop the unsafer encounter. While the individualistic approach may not afford as "accurate" a representation of what actually occurred in the encounter as interviewing both sexual partners would, individual interviews do provide enough information for the person to think about what he needs to do in order to change his behavior if he so chooses.

Media Campaigns: Guilt, Self-efficacy, and Positive Reinforcement

"I felt so ashamed and guilty," Phil confessed in chapter 4. "I keep promising myself that it will never, ever happen again." I am not the first to discover the internalization of shame and guilt by those who break the safer sex social norm. Walt Odets (1995) argues that gay men have always felt shame and guilt for their homosexual behaviors, and today, given the moral push for safer sex, gay men now feel guilty for having had such an experience.

Health education has continued to drive home a safer sex norm, sometimes in a subtle fashion but at other times in a destructive manner. In 1995 the City of West Hollywood and the Gay and Lesbian Community Services Center (GLCSC) launched an abrasive "in your face" health campaign, consisting of eleven billboards printed with bold, stark white letters against a black background. The text read: YOUR FRIENDS ARE DEAD. DEMAND SAFER SEX NOW. In its regular public relations publication mailed out to West Hollywood residents, the city touted these obtrusive billboards as "a bold, new advertising campaign . . . expressing the reality and consequence of unsafe sexual behavior . . . [and] designed to be a wake-up call for the community by encouraging discussions that will lead to safer sexual behavior" (*City News*, September 1995).

As if this campaign were not offensive enough, the Los Angeles GLCSC also launched another ad campaign featuring graphic pictures of people in the last stages of AIDS. The supporters of this campaign believed that too many "positive," "glamorous," and attractive images of people infected with HIV have dominated the media. They wanted to show people "what the disease really is." They feared that some gay men, particularly younger gay men, connected being HIV-infected with having good looks because of the supposedly "glamorous images" portrayed of the HIV-infected (Simmons 1995).

Gay men, especially in the thirty to forty-four age group, having suffered an enormous loss in this epidemic, know all too well that their friends are dead—with many other friends still in the process of dying. They have seen the graphic end stages of AIDS in person and face-to-face. They know firsthand "what the disease really is." Gay men are already all too aware of HIV, its consequences, and basic AIDS 101 facts.

Such insensitive tactics can only increase guilt, not overcome it— not to mention the impact such messages are bound to have on people already living with and struggling against HIV infection (see Turner 1995). These campaigns were in poor taste at best, and at worst, injurious. We can only hope that negative advertising campaigns do not push gay men downward into feelings of hopelessness.

Out of frustration and with the best of intentions (lest we forget the road to hell), educators in other cities have resorted to similar tactics. In 1993 the San Francisco AIDS Foundation developed a media campaign based upon the slogan, "The Moral Majority is made up of . . . men who express their sexuality in a healthy way" (in Odets 1995). Such approaches in effect question the morality of gay men, like the men in this book, who have occasional slips, while pushing them further and further into the closet. But coming out of the closet as someone who occasionally has unsafer sex is yet another important step, and this will only occur in a safer environment free of initial judgment.

At any rate, for this group of gay men, media campaigns will probably have little or no influence in changing their behaviors toward a healthier direction. Media campaigns are best used to make an impact in awareness, or in basic knowledge and attitudes, and cannot, by themselves, change behaviors (Rice and Atkin 1989).

Media campaigns may successfully be used, however, as a form of positive reinforcement—not for *always* practicing safer sex but for practicing it most of the time. Gay men have accomplished a necessary degree of behavioral change that other groups have not, and for this they should be congratulated. The Gay Men's Health Crisis (GMHC) in New York City put out a positive reinforcement pamphlet called *Keep It Up!* with a photo of two happy, smiling, and sexy shirtless young men. More such pamphlets would be useful as long as their producers do not assume that gay men are practicing safer sex all the time, but instead emphasize that gay men have made perhaps a historically unprecedented change in sexual behavior.

My experience with health educators, epidemiologists, psychologists, and other professionals tells me that they are afraid to adopt such an approach. They are concerned that individuals may take this message and assume that it is okay to have occasional unsafer sex. It is true that some may internalize reinforcement messages in this way, but the consequences of not switching approaches may be even worse. If you are in doubt, turn back and read the stories in the previous chapters. Read them closely, paying particular attention to the men's feelings of guilt and shame after an unsafer encounter, reticent feelings buried in their private thoughts.

As I have already stated in previous chapters, guilt may have a negative impact over time if it is not dealt with in a more positive fashion. In response to his guilt, for instance, a gay man who currently practices safer sex most of the time may eventually feel that he is no longer capable of practicing safer sex at all or give it up altogether. In social psychology and health education this feeling is often referred to as a lowered self-efficacy. Self-efficacy is an individual's perception about how capable he or she is in performing some health-related behavior (Bandura 1977, 1986). Self-efficacy is not a permanent characteristic but changes through time and situation based upon cumulative experience. It is fuzzy in that, in some situations, a person may feel greater self-efficacy than in others. It is dynamic in that a degree of self-efficacy may contribute to a safer sex experience and, at the same time, is impacted by that experience as well as by previous experiences. Unfortunately, media campaigns like the ones I have described can lower self-efficacy by encouraging a gay man to doubt his "morality" and fostering feelings of guilt and shame.

There is no full-proof method of health education or psychosocial intervention, but some interventions may be better than others. Finding an optimal strategy should be the goal. In addition to media campaigns, removing the social gags from gay men's sexual feelings and experiences is another piece of this strategy, and professionally run or peer-run groups can provide facilitation for this disclosure. "Unprotected sex is commonplace among gay men," says Odets, "and unless it can be talked about rather than merely prohibited, there will be no opportunity for making relatively clear, conscious decisions about it" (1995:181).

But taking action, not just talking about unsafer sex, is also necessary, both in impacting contextual self-efficacy and in changing and maintaining a higher frequency of condom use or other less risky sexual behaviors. Many gay men do want to learn ways to better manage their sexual behaviors, and to adopt ways to reduce their risk. Interventions that allow for individual motivation, individual choice, and individual actions that foster social support, and that take a nonpathological approach by recognizing that the desire for unsafer sex is a natural, evolved human drive may be more effective than those that push safer sex within the vague rubric of morality. A drive for sexual pleasure is not something to feel guilty about, but instead is something that can be managed.

Workshops: Communication and Situational Factors

Sexual communication, I have argued, begins at first sight, when two men lock eye contact. Their eyes dilate, and one man may wink or provide some other nonverbal signal of sexual interest. They may simply hold a stare longer than a casual glance. One or both partners will signal interest. When Johnny had his unsafer experience outside of his relationship with Ralph, his young provocateur signaled his sexual interest by standing close to Johnny as they both browsed pornography in a book store.

Once interest is established, conversation eventually occurs, perhaps focusing on small talk, or in some contexts the two men proceed directly to crotch-groping and erotic talk. In the age of cyberspace, even body presence is not essential. Roger began his sexual ritual on the Internet, communicating with his unsafer partner disembodied.

Although nonverbal and verbal communication mainly sets the sexual stage, sometimes this communication also distinguishes sexual roles (top versus bottom, for example) and fires up the first neuronal sparks of sexual arousal. However, among gay men there is rarely or never a discussion about specific sexual acts and their safety. Not one of these men discussed safer sex with their partner before plunging into erotic foreplay and sex. They expected the sexual meeting to be safer, not to be an encounter ending in unprotected anal intercourse. In their minds, what else would it be but safer sex? Gay men tend to expect their partner to abide by the norm even if they themselves have had occasional slips.

Communication before foreplay, when arousal is in its early stages and rationality has not been too compromised, may help prevent some unsafer sex events, so that increasing one's sexual communication skills may help reduce unsafer sex encounters. Increasing these skills requires practice and is best done in a one-on-one or small group intervention (Kelly et al. 1989; Kelly 1995).

Even if safer sex communication is incorporated into the ritual of sexual partner selection, several other pleasure-inducing situational factors that I have described with the help of those interviewed may still lead a man into heightened arousal, to become "caught in the moment." Given that these factors vary greatly across individuals, a more individualized approach might be of greater assistance in reducing risk. In one such method, the individual identifies his situational "triggers" to heightened arousal and develops techniques for controlling his responses to them. This type of intervention is sometimes called self-behavior modification or self-management (Kelly 1995; Watson and Tharp 1989).

Just as with the development of communication skills, self-behavior modification is best when used as an individual or small group technique, but it cannot be completed in a one-time workshop (Kelly et al. 1989; Kelly 1995; Watson and Tharp 1989). This intervention method requires multisessions so that the individual can acquire skills over time by analyzing slips when they occur and then by making the most effective modifications and developing successful strategies based upon self-analyses. It works best when the behavior is still a rarity, as it is for the gay men here—in other words, when the unsafer behaviors are merely an early warning sign (Schunk and Carbonari 1984).

According to Kanfer (1970, 1971, 1980), the self-behavior "regulation" or modification process is made up of at least three components (but keep in mind that these components are fuzzy and overlap). Kanfer's three components are self-monitoring, self-evaluation, and self-reinforcement. Self-monitoring and self-evaluation are used to analyze one's triggers to unsafer and safer encounters and to maintain a record of one's attempts to reduce the number of unsafer experiences. Self-reinforcement involves taking action based upon the results of self-monitoring and self-evaluation.

In self-behavior monitoring and self-evaluation, each individual self-analyzes his safer/unsafer sex behaviors (and fantasies), perhaps by way of comparison and contrasts, in order to determine what ignites his heightened arousal and unsafer sex. These triggers generally include—but are not limited to—such domains as the partner's physical characteristics and/or sexual abilities, the environment, interactive sensory stimulation, and sexual accessories. These I outlined in the last chapter.

On account of the importance of individual variation within these domains, each man must identify his own specific triggers. For example, he may ask himself, "What specific characteristics about my unsafer partner were different from those of safer partners? What are my fantasy sexual acts, places, and men, and how do they relate to my safer and unsafer sex experiences? What is it about the place where I met my unsafer partner and where we had sex that might be related to my fantasy or different from my safer sex encounters?" It is these types of self-probing questions that help a man to develop a keen self-awareness of what might lead to an unsafer sexual experience.

For some, this exercise may also include serious reflection on their thoughts and emotions during the unsafer encounter. Gold (1995) has already demonstrated the value that taking this kind of introspective inventory can have to help gay men reduce, if not completely eliminate, their number of unsafer slips—a worthy and realistic goal.

Once these triggers have been identified, the next step is to develop techniques for preventing unsafer slips as often as possible. These techniques will make up the program participant's plan of self-reinforcement. Bob in chapter 3 provides a good example of how self-reinforcement might be carried out. When a sexual situation begins to unfold and he feels the interaction may be getting "out of control," he has trained himself to turn on "a little voice" in his head to tell him to slow down.

Still, just as with self-evaluation and self-monitoring, self-reinforcement methods will not be the same for everyone. Each individual must develop his own technique or strategy, one that works for him. If strategy *A* does not work, he can develop strategy *B* and even strategy *C* until he finds one or more that help him gain greater control, at least most of the time.

He can participate in small group or one-on-one guided practice sessions in which he acts out different potential strategies (Kelly 1995). At the same time, he may decide that it is worthwhile to avoid self-identified "higher-risk" situations (if not sex), at least for the short run (Kelly et al. 1989, 1990a, 1990b; Miller 1995). Avoidance is unlikely to be beneficial over the long haul, but he can reintroduce himself to higher-risk situations over time once he has developed new risk-reduction strategies (Schunk and Carbonari 1984).

In time, attempts at safer sex should be encouraged, not condemned. By way of attempts followed by positive reinforcement, an individual's self-efficacy will be further increased as he ventures out into his sexual world. Some change is better than none, and a little change, if handled appropriately, can lead to more change. After all, further successful attempts may not come easily since the adoption of a new approach or behavior is bound to hit snags in the early stages of acquisition. If the individual attributes the problem to his ability to use condoms at all, then he will likely perceive a lower self-efficacy and thus "relapse" into unsafer behaviors (Brownell et al. 1986; Marlatt and Gordon 1985). Thus, framing a slip as a failure instead of a natural process in behavior management could lead to the very situation that health educators want most to prevent: the individual's total and complete abandonment of condoms.

Gay men also need to learn to set realistic goals. Goals should be small and quickly attainable, with built-in rewards (Schunk and Carbonari 1984). Instead of goals such as "I will not have unsafer sex over the next six months," a more appropriate goal might be "I will discuss safer sex with the next guy I pick up before we go to bed." In Jerry's case of bingeing and purging, the goal may be to attend one session with a therapist to discuss his high level of sexual fear; and for the couple, Johnny and Ralph, it may be that Johnny will call or see Ralph whenever he feels pangs to sleep around. The point is that each goal is a step in the process of self-reinforcement and ultimately to risk reduction. If unsafer sex occurs, a reevaluation of the situational factors and / or sexual triggers as well as of the coping strategy itself is in order.

In the United States, both Gay Men's Health Crisis in New York City and AIDS Project Los Angeles (APLA) have developed programs based upon self-behavior modification. GMHC's program, "Keep It Up" (of which the pamphlet mentioned earlier is a part), is designed to "enhance competencies in several areas and includes: identification of what practices participants consider risky, social support mobilization techniques, high-risk situation analysis, identification of rationalizations for unsafe sex and barriers to safer sex, coping with rationalizations for safer sex, confidence building, and verbal commitments to safer sex" (Miller 1995).

Unfortunately, "Keep It Up" is a one-shot workshop; and (at least in theory) it also preaches condoms for oral sex. By taking such a stance, the program does not appear to embrace unprotected oral sex as a risk-reduction strategy. (This assumption is based upon the Miller article cited above and below.) Furthermore, evaluation of the program's effectiveness is at best uncertain since 90 percent of the 202 workshop participants who attended between May 1991 to February 1993 reported that they did not engage in unprotected anal intercourse before attending the workshop and at follow-up interviews (Miller 1995:59).

APLA has a similar program called "Sex Essentials." The intervention has a monthly magazine (or "zine" as they call it), which discusses a range of topics related to safer sex, gay relationships, and other issues such as death and dying. The zine also advertises safer sex workshops, flashes many provocative pictures of sexy shirtless men, compares and contrasts brands of condoms, and even provides critiques of gay pornographic films.

Most striking are some of the zine's advertisements, used by APLA to promote the agency's own "Sex Essentials" safer sex workshops and utilizing catchy slogans such as BE A PUSHY BOTTOM and SAFER SEX SUCKS. The former jingle acknowledges that practicing safer sex all the time is not the real behavioral norm among gay men while the latter taps into the authentic feelings that safer sex is not the most pleasurable sex. By using a condom, the catchphrase concedes, gay men are sacrificing some degree of physical and psychological

pleasure. In some advertisements, the health educators have provided statistics about the men who attend their workshop, including
the main reasons given by participants for having unsafer sex. (By
the way, the top two reasons given by their workshop participants
were the same as those found in my qualitative interviews: being
with a lover or significant other and being caught in the heat of the
moment.) These lucid statistics communicate to a potential workshop participant that he is not the only gay man in the sexual universe with these experiences and feelings.

All of APLA's advertisements are directed exclusively toward
anal sex without a condom. Even the full-page ad featuring SAFER SEX
SUCKS (alluding to oral sex) in large white letters continues with the
following: "It's hard work and not easy. But you're worth it. Using a
latex condom during anal sex will substantially reduce the risk of
HIV transmission" (AIDS Project Los Angeles 1995). The ad does not
push the use of a condom "every time" and acknowledges that risk
reduction is no minor task and does not occur at the snap of a finger.

Woefully, however, the zine appears to be slanted to a younger
gay male population than to an "older" cohort of men (such as those
interviewed in this book). Expanding the magazine to include issues
of concern for older gay men or developing another one specifically
for gay men thirty and over could be a tremendous help to this
group. As Alexander, the HIV-negative AIDS service provider
pointed out, there is little available for HIV-negative men his age. In
any case, APLA's zine is a substantial improvement over such mis-
guided efforts as YOUR FRIENDS ARE DEAD.

In addition to using the zine as a form of educational outreach,
APLA volunteers take to the streets of West Hollywood and recruit
gay men into the workshops. There are three APLA-administered
"Sex Essentials" workshops. The first workshop, "Latex, Lube, and
Beyond," explores "the latest in latex love, risk reduction, and offers
opportunities to discover options for enhancing our sexual experiences" (AIDS Project Los Angeles 1995). The intervention is designed
for those men who need to learn or gain reinforcement of safer sex
knowledge, attitudes, beliefs, and behaviors.

The second workshop, "Understanding Ourselves," is a self-
behavior modification workshop in which participants "discuss
what influences our sexual decisions and how we can change unfa-

vorable situations to more successful encounters" (AIDS Project Los Angeles 1995). The last workshop component is an "HIV Negative Men's Discussion Forum," which includes monthly discussions of topics such as "Dating Someone Who is HIV Positive," "Surviving Loss," and "HIV Negative and Feeling Guilty." Ideally, the forums allow men to share their experiences with each other in an open and supportive environment.

In 1994 I attended the pilot workshop of the "Sex Essentials" program, which at that time had only one type of meeting, but it has changed and evolved (as it should) over time. So in December 1995, I went again to the self-behavior modification workshop, "Understanding Ourselves." Although "Understanding Ourselves" is supposedly targeted to younger gay men, the ten men who attended that Wednesday evening covered an age spectrum ranging from about twenty-five to forty years of age and represented diverse ethnic groups. Ten may sound like a small number, but it was actually a good turnout, given that Los Angeles was having its first rain in nine months, the first rain of winter. And in any case, this type of intervention is best with smaller groups.

Five of the attendees appeared to be Caucasian, two African-American, and the remaining three were Asian-American. As might be expected when a group of strangers come together for the first time, the ten men were slow to get started but soon loosened up and shared their thoughts and feelings throughout the two-hour workshop, both in smaller groups of three or four and also with the entire group.

The main volunteer facilitator was a forty-eight-year-old lesbian, not a gay man, and I think this may have contributed to the reluctance of some to discuss sexual issues in a more graphic manner. The room was bright and stark. Folding chairs were arranged in a semi-circle to create a more open social space and to encourage conversation, but the setting was not very intimate. One participant commented to me afterward that he would have preferred to have had the workshop in a person's home, a more comfortable setting that is more conducive "to talking about something as intimate as sex."

Despite these environmental limitations, many of the men did reveal some intimate details about themselves. Among other things, participants were asked to come up with reasons for having sex in general. Four men—the two African-Americans and two Caucasians—

immediately, and with much enthusiasm, called out answers and came up with an extensive list. Not surprisingly, the reasons cited for the most part were emotional and situational: mood, desire, habit (one of the participants said "instinct," but the facilitator wrote "habit"), pleasure, circumstances, drugs and alcohol, and spontaneity.

The group concocted additional lists for "triggers" to not using a condom. The most agreed-upon was "caught in the heat of the moment." As one participant described the heat of the moment, "It's as if my thoughts follow my body, not the other way around . . . when the guy is extra physically attractive." Another man blurted out, "natural instinct"— a different man from before—and a couple of the others nodded, but an uneasy silence retarded the flow of conversation. After glancing around the semicircle for a moment, this same man reprimanded himself with "I guess that's just an excuse." I leaned back into my chair, frustrated and sad, suppressing my impatience to explore this area further. The facilitator moved on, ignoring his response, and erased the hush with the scribble of her magic marker as it listed other, more acceptable, reasons across her large notepad.

At one point, there was an interactive discussion, interrupted with giggles and laughter, about what "a pain" condoms are to use. "They don't tell you on the package that these things are difficult to open," said one of the participants with words reminiscent of those used by Jerry in chapter 7, "and the lube gets messy. It's a real production and a lot of work."

Although no one had suggested "self-esteem" as a reason to have unsafer sex, the facilitator at least once or twice attempted to link many men's explanations to this psychological construct *du jour*. This move was lamentable as the men were being honest and were attending this workshop to make sense of their individual difficulties in maintaining safer sex, not for a diagnosis. I did notice, however, that when she asked the men if they agreed, there was a silent pause and heads did not nod in agreement; but I still remember thinking as I stared at their flushed faces, "I'm sure they doubt their worth now if they didn't before."

In spite of the facilitator-related problems in the program's delivery on that particular evening, the workshop, according to the men attending—and I agree—was of tremendous value. Throughout the workshop, the men learned behavior-modification skills. They mastered visualization techniques in which they recalled the "who, what, when, where, and how" of their last sexual experience and other details about the day in which it happened. As each man lifted his eyes from his personal sexual visualization, he immediately recorded his virtual memory in a small logbook which he would take with him at the evening's end. The men were taught how to read patterns in their sexual lives, to understand why they take sexual risks. And of most import, as one of the African-American participants shared, "Tonight I learned that others have my same feelings. I am not alone." Others bobbed their heads in apparent agreement.

At the workshop's end, the facilitator repeated the program's pragmatic and meritorious goals: "to use condoms more consistently and to reduce one's risk." What a breath of fresh air! It was startling not to hear the less practical goal, "to use a condom every single time." One of the men cocked his head to the right and squinted as if it were the first time he had heard such a fuzzy goal.

After I walked away from the meeting and concluded a brief conversation with one of the participants, I returned to my car, flipped on the map light, and scribbled a few memory-jogging field notes in my own "Sex Essentials" logbook. I made a note about how advantageous it would be to provide follow-up workshops in which the men could bring their personal logbooks and, with one-on-one assistance, form an intervention plan, which would then be revised on an ongoing basis as the fluid, ever-changing areas of sexual experience complicated (while simultaneously improving) the best-laid plan.

Even though I have argued that it is doubtful that a one-shot self-behavior modification workshop will have a long-lasting impact, it is still too early to determine the true effectiveness of the "Sex Essentials" program in maintaining or in improving safer sex behaviors. The program's evaluators are currently recruiting a group of seventy-five men to follow over a one-year period to assess the program's behavioral results. This should provide some strong evaluative data even though the design is not an experimental one. I here want to caution the program's administrators (as well as the administrators of similar programs) not to measure their program's success based upon all-or-nothing criteria such as consistent versus inconsistent condom use or to consider their program ineffective if the level of risk behaviors is maintained rather than decreased (Miller 1995). Preventing an *increase* in the frequency of unprotected sex is just as meaningful as decreasing or eliminating the number of unsafer encounters. Finally, the programs should not only target unsafer anal sex but also consider that those individuals whose strategy has been to cut down their frequency of unprotected anal sex by replacing this with unprotected oral sex as indeed having taken measures to reduce their risk.

After all is said and done, this type of intervention is a *process* and thus may hamper gay men's giving up of unsafer sex altogether while, at the same time, it may decrease the frequency of their unsafer risk-taking behaviors. But even if educators, other health professionals, and gay men do follow these proscriptive methods as outlined, some individuals will undoubtedly have one or more, but potentially rare, unsafer encounters in their sexual lifetimes. Hopefully such events will be the spur to motivation for further action and not experienced as guilt-inducing events. Moreover, not every gay man will want to invest the effort and time required for the ongoing process of maintaining safer sex behaviors (Miller 1995) and will continue to practice unsafer sex at least occasionally.

These likely probabilities are sometimes disheartening to health educators frozen in binary time/space and locked in their prison of all-or-nothing outcomes. Yet if most gay men do not consistently practice safer sex, does this mean that health education has failed? Should health educators give up? Absolutely not. At the population-at-risk level, if most people practice safer sex most of the time, then a high degree of success will indeed have been achieved. Individuals will have reduced their chances of becoming infected and rates of new infections will be reduced. Just as medical doctors have acknowledged that a cure is not around the corner and that their best available approach is to manage the disease, perhaps health educators, psychologists, and others involved in HIV prevention need to learn to manage the epidemic and to stop berating themselves for not having eliminated it.

Back to Evolution

Public health efforts have actually only eradicated one infectious disease—smallpox—and the situation for smallpox was very different than that for HIV. Although the smallpox virus was spread by touch or through respiration (rather than through bodily fluids and sexual contact), cases were easily identified and people were infectious for only four or five days (Garrett 1994). With HIV, a person may not even know that he or she is infected for quite some time and can unknowingly pass the infection on to a partner for a time period much longer than four or five days.

In the 1960s, when the World Health Organization (WHO) launched a smallpox eradication campaign, there was already a cheap and effective vaccine available, a vaccine developed by Edward Jenner in 1796. Jenner observed that milkmaids afflicted with cowpox, a less virulent, smallpox-like disease transmitted by cows, were not likely to come down with smallpox. Based upon this observation alone, he inoculated an eight-year-old boy with cowpox and, six weeks later, injected him with pus from smallpox. He was successful. Although the boy was mildly affected by the cowpox, he did not show any manifestations of smallpox (Biddle 1995).

For Jenner and his "subject," there was no informed consent mandated. Likewise, during the WHO smallpox eradication campaign, when health workers uncovered a case of smallpox, they isolated or quarantined the afflicted person and vaccinated everyone in the surrounding area, sometimes against their will and of course without an informed consent (Garrett 1994). In contemporary times, to do this type of experiment or intervention with HIV would be unethical and impossible, and though I agree with a more ethical form of HIV prevention, ethics do slow the race for an effective vaccine. Luckily though, from an evolutionary perspective, it is not necessary to eliminate HIV transmission, just to reduce it. Therefore, draconian measures are *probably* unnecessary.

In the preceding chapter, I spent a great deal of time discussing evolution in the context of human adaptation to HIV as part of a novel environment, but that is only half the story. We are not the only organism adapting to environmental change. HIV is also changing and adapting to its environment, of which human beings are a part. In brief, HIV itself evolves. When human beings change their behavior, some strains or future strains of HIV will be better adapted to this change than others. This is not just a quirk of HIV but is standard for most microbes.

Natural selection for microbes such as bacteria and viruses occurs in two ways: within host and between host. *Host* refers to a person who is infected by a given microbe. "Within host" selection occurs as our immune system or a new medication successfully eliminates the less adaptive microbial strains which have infected our bodies. This leaves the more adapted strains behind to survive and reproduce (Lappé 1995; Neese and Williams 1994). Thus each time researchers develop a new AIDS "bullet" (in the form of antiretrovirals commonly identified by their abbreviated names of AZT, DDI, DDC, D3T, and more recent sophisticated bullets such as protease inhibitors—and the list is certain to grow), the virus mutates and becomes resistant, or the medication is not effective against all existing viral variations. There is variation, in other words, in the ability of each virus to survive and reproduce (Garrett 1994; Lappé 1995; Neese and Williams 1994).

Sadly, a virus like HIV replicates rapidly by human standards and can produce several generations in a relatively short period of time. (By contrast, it takes human beings at least nine months to produce and years to raise just one or more offspring.) The more rapid the reproduction, the greater the mutation rate, which means that the virus mutates in a rather rapid fashion. These new mutant strains may be more adapted to their medicated environment than were their "ancestors." The mutant variants will have resistance. In a nutshell, adaptation occurs when the more resistant strains of HIV are able to survive the medication and to reproduce.

"Within host" selection may also favor more or less virulent strains of a microbe when humans do not take their treatments full term. In the case of tuberculosis, for example, some individuals for various reasons do not complete their six-month-to-one-year regimen of drugs and discontinue use after a month or two when outward symptoms have dissipated. When this occurs, the drug has killed only the least resistant and less virulent strains of the tuberculosis-causing bacillus, leaving behind the more resistant and virulent bacillus to reproduce. Thus today there exists a more dangerous and resistant form of tuberculosis, multiple drug resistant (MDR) tuberculosis (Garrett 1994; Lappé 1995).

At the same time that "within host" selection is occurring, "between host" selection, much more hopeful for controlling viral strain selection, is also taking place. "Between host" selection is related to transmission (which for HIV, I will demonstrate shortly, is dependent upon behavior change). Microbes must transmit themselves to continue replication (reproduction). Those microbes that successfully transmit themselves are more likely to survive and reproduce. Within the theory of natural selection, they have greater "reproductive success."

Furthermore, a microbe's ability to transmit itself is intrinsically linked with its degree of virulence. During "between host" selection, more or less virulent strains are selected depending upon the mode and difficulty of microbe transmission (Ewald 1994; Neese and Williams 1994). For a ready example before turning to HIV, consider malaria as contrasted with the common cold. Malaria is caused by a genus of protozoans called plasmodium and is spread by way of a biological vector, the female *Anopheles* mosquito. Once the pesky mosquito sucks its sanguine diet from a new host, leaving the plasmodium traveler behind, the new host becomes extremely ill, is bedridden with soaring fevers, and may even die. Plasmodium is a virulent microbe—virulent because it does not need to rely upon its host (you or me) for transmission. The host does not have to feel well for the malaria-causing microbe to be successful at finding another host. The ailing patient can just lie there, feverish and delusional, as the mosquito sucks up his or her plasmodium-rich blood. Once nourished, the mosquito flies away seeking another victim, thus spreading the infection from host to host. The mosquito does all the work, so plasmodium can be highly virulent, widely spread, and reproductively successful (Biddle 1995; Ewald 1994; Lappé 1995; Neese and Williams 1994).

In contrast, the rhinovirus which causes the common cold is of low virulence. It relies upon human mobility for transmission. We have to feel well enough to go to school, the office, or the grocery store—sneezing, wheezing, coughing, and wiping our noses, thus expelling the virus onto money and other things, as well as other people—for the virus to come into contact with new hosts to infect (Biddle 1995; Ewald 1994; Garrett 1994; Neese and Williams 1994). The less virulent the rhinovirus, the more likely the host will get out and about, and thus the greater likelihood of transmission. Those less virulent strains that allow the infected person to mingle, so to speak, amidst the rest of the human population are more likely to be transmitted than are the more debilitating ones and thus will have increased reproductive success.

Unlike plasmodium and the rhinovirus, the mode of transmission for HIV is primarily, though not exclusively, by way of sex, and sex requires a certain amount of human energy to seek out sexual partners and to perform sexual acts. Because of this transmission mode, the host has to be kept alive and feeling well for at least some time until transmission to a new host is likely to take place. Once in the new host, the virus can go on replicating itself.

Reducing the frequency of unsafer sex decreases the likelihood of infection from the human's point of view, but it also reduces the likelihood of transmission from the "perspective" of the virus. The lesser the probability of transmission, the greater the reproductive success of the less virulent strains. Those viral strains that kill or incapacitate their host before transmission die out and do not continue on. Thus if the frequency of unsafer sex is reduced in a population, the less virulent strains should be selected for and have a higher probability of transmission (i.e., to survive and reproduce).

Put another way, if most people use condoms most of the time, the probable length of time between a person's HIV exposure and the opportunity for HIV transmission will on average be lengthened, and only those strains that keep the host healthy for a greater length of time will get their chance to infect and continue replication.

On the flip side, if a greater frequency of unprotected sex is occurring within a population, then the more virulent HIV strains, which also replicate much faster once inside the host, will be more easily and rapidly transmitted. The host does not have to be kept alive for very long before the microbe will have the opportunity to be passed on, infecting another host and continuing its replication in its new human territory. In the bluntest of terms, the more deadly strains will have greater reproductive success than the less virulent, more people will be potentially infected, and those infected will conceivably die more rapidly (Ewald 1994; Lappé 1995; Neese and Williams 1994).

Don't forget—on a brighter note—that reducing HIV transmission (not necessarily eliminating it) can select for less virulent viral strains that keep those who do get infected alive longer. As Marc Lappé points out:

As the opportunity for transmission drops with diminished contagious sexual contacts, only those disease-causing organisms that have
delayed onset and relatively mild manifestations are selected.... Only
by *slowing the rate* of transmission of this deadly disease will the virus
[HIV] be encouraged to evolve toward longer latent periods and clin-
icians be given the breathing room they need to develop more effective
treatments. (1995:113, emphasis added; also see Ewald 1994)

Thus managing the epidemic may reduce harm not only to those
who do not become infected but also to those who do as HIV evolves
and adapts to human behavioral change. Paul Ewald (1994), an evolutionary biologist, has argued that such a selective/adaptive course
is already occurring among HIV strains found among gay men, an
evolutionary path that I truly hope we and HIV will continue to take.

I have zealously argued that all-or-nothing approaches which
ignore the evolved and ambiguous sexual realities of everyday life
(as so eloquently expressed by the men in this book) will not reduce
transmission of HIV, but indeed may increase it by enforcing and
reinforcing guilt and a lack of self-efficacy with each and every slip;
moreover, as a grand and fatal finality, such approaches give more
virulent HIV strains a helping hand. Therefore, in one last plea, let
me drive home the point that reducing transmission—not eliminating transmission—is truly our only hope at this stage of the epidemic. To realize this feat is no small endeavor and would be the
noblest of accomplishments. But it requires the pragmatic and stead-
fast efforts of individuals, communities, professionals, and governmental agencies; and further, any such endeavor must consider the
amorphous and unpredictable world of sexual pleasure, a fuzzy
world to which HIV has so well adapted.

If we are wise enough to view the world as it really is, as a fuzzy
world, we can learn to see how the big picture and the little picture
connect in the overall scheme of things—where daily human experience is acted out and pleasure is savored, where viruses may evolve
but human behavior can be changed, and yes, where people, including gay men, sometimes have sex without a condom, but then try to
do better.

Appendix A

Methodology

Reliability and Validity

In my research I attempted to address reliability and validity to the extent possible with qualitative methods. Qualitative methods have very strong validity but not necessarily strong reliability. Nevertheless, some anthropologists and other qualitative researchers attempt to increase reliability by using a variety of data collection methods (Kirk and Miller 1988; Pelto and Pelto 1978). Others attempt to combine qualitative and quantitative methods (Pelto and Pelto 1978) and/or to document ethnographic decision-making (Kirk and Miller 1988).

I strove to increase reliability and replicability without the loss of construct validity by the use of more than one data collection method—i.e., participant observation, interviews, life histories, and focus groups. Second, I made an attempt to present all the information necessary to replicate the project by presenting data with corresponding method of collection (see Turner 1994). However, this does not mean that I was able to achieve the strength of combining qualitative and quantitative methods in the use of qualitative methods alone.

Participant Observation

Participant observation differs from observation in that the researcher learns and collects information by participating in the activities and/or behaviors being observed (Spradley 1980). Participation is helpful in exploring the emic or "insider" perspective (Pelto and Pelto 1978). In his classic 1922 work *Argonauts of the Western Pacific*, Bronislaw Malinowski refers to participation in day-to-day and ritualistic activities as "learning how to behave" like a native (1961:7).

Spradley (1980) differentiates participant observation into four types based upon the researcher's level of participation. The four types are passive, moderate, active, and complete. It is important that the researcher be up-front and clear about his or her level of participation for the sake of methodological rigor. The type of participation may depend upon the phenomenon or activity under study.

The first data collection method used in this project was participant observation. According to Spradley, "The participant observer comes to a social situation with two purposes: (1) to engage in activities appropriate to the situation and (2) to observe the activities, people, and physical aspects of the situation" (1980:54). Part of my research is based upon my experiences living in West Hollywood since the beginning of January 1993 until January 1996 as well as upon conversations with key informants. In this case, I was a complete participant. Also per Spradley (1980), complete participation occurs when the opportunistic researcher decides to study an activity in which he or she already participates.

I also did participant observation by attending at least one prevention workshop targeting gay men at AIDS Project Los Angeles (APLA) and another at the Los Angeles Gay and Lesbian Community Services Center (GLCSC). Issues about practicing safer sex and not practicing safer sex were discussed by the groups in both workshops, and the men who attended were self-identified as having difficulties maintaining safer sex behaviors. I had never attended either workshop before, although I had developed an evaluation for the program at APLA, where I was employed until March 1993.

My level of participation varied with each workshop. For the workshop at APLA, my participation was passive. In passive participation, the researcher plays the role of a bystander, loiterer, or spectator (Spradley 1980). This type of participation was appropriate to the activity as this workshop did not consist of compulsory group activities (which would have required me to be involved at a more intensive level of participation). Therefore I could be a passive participant without greatly disturbing the natural flow of the setting.

In the second workshop, I was both a moderate participant and an active participant, depending upon the workshop activity. Some activities were compulsory and required body touching and ritual participation. In these activities, I was an active participant in order to maintain workshop flow and to understand the impact of these experiences on the participants. In moderate participation, the researcher balances observation and participation, while in active participation the researcher does what other people are doing (Spradley 1980).

In addition to providing descriptive data, the data collected from these workshops were used to develop an interview guide to gather further information in one-on-one interviews. For the purpose of this book, I participated in the APLA program again in December 1995 (see chapter 9).

Interviews

Like participant observation, interviews are also used to explore the emic or "insider" perspective. Interviews capture feelings, emotions, attitudes, and what people say they do (Pelto and Pelto 1978), but there is often a discrepancy between what people actually do and what they say they do. This is one of the major problems associated with interviews and is often problematic in studies of sexual behavior, particularly if discussions about sexual behaviors are considered to be culturally and socially taboo (Coyle, Boruch, and Turner 1991).

However, based upon interviews with gay and lesbian youth in Chicago, Herdt and Boxer (1991) note that the quality—validity—of interviews about sexual behaviors can be increased by matching the interviewer on gender, age, race, and sexual identity with the interviewee. This was important, according to the researchers, since "many of these youth are reluctant to discuss their lives with those who are heterosexually identified" (175). But the authors caution against using this method as a panacea for all cross-cultural work.

In this project the interviewer—myself—was matched with the interviewees in that I am a Caucasian gay man between the ages of thirty and forty-four and resided for the year during the study in the community of West Hollywood. This strategy may have improved the validity of the responses, but there may still be a difference in what people say they do and what they do, particularly in regard to sexual behaviors that cannot be cross-checked by direct observation.

Just as there is more than one type of participant observation, there is also more than one type of qualitative interview. Bauman et al. (1992) distinguish between several types of interviews. At least two are relevant to this project: (1) the in-depth unstructured, unstandardized interview, and (2) the structured in-depth interview.

The in-depth unstructured, unstandardized interview contains no predefined set of questions or topics and imposes no order upon the flow of information. Respondents are encouraged to talk about a topic that the researcher has selected, but the specific themes, areas, and orders of discussion are completely determined by the respondent (Bauman et al. 1992). This method is similar to conversation and may take place anywhere at any opportunistic moment or place, such as a market or even a door stoop (Briggs 1984; Scrimshaw and Hurtado 1987). These types of interviews may be used when no preliminary method such as participant observation has been used, or to supplement other methods, and/or when little is known abut the phenomenon under study.

In contrast, the structured in-depth interview capitalizes on the richness of qualitative open-ended responses but structures the content of the interview through the use of an interview guide. This ensures that the same information is gathered from each interviewee. Although this interview requires specific data from all respondents, it is flexible in the order of interview topics and the wording of questions and probes (Bauman et al. 1992; Scrimshaw 1990).

Interview guides were constructed based upon participant observation in the intervention programs of APLA and GLCSC .

Life Histories

In addition to observation, participant observation, and interviews, I also collected more extensive personal documents on a given single individual by way of collecting a life history. Life histories offer vivid and rich information about the life passages of individuals (Pelto and Pelto 1978).

The validity of life history data, just as with the validity of interviews in general, has been criticized as being difficult to check against observed behaviors (Pelto and Pelto 1978). However, Langness (1965) argues that the patterns of people's beliefs and perceptions are more important than factual behaviors.

The purpose of the life history for this project was less for determining factual behaviors and more for uncovering perceptions of life events that contributed to the individual's perception of behaviors. In doing the life history, I tried a unique methodological approach. Since the population that I studied is a literate one, I asked the informant to write his life history. This written history was used by me during the interviews as a guide (i.e., the person did not have it in front of him). If the informant's oral history deviated at any time from the written one, the contradiction, or the perceived contradiction, was discussed.

The life history provides context—along with the community ethnography—for better understanding the complexity of "relapse" into unsafe sex for this group of men. Furthermore, as with participant observation, it was helpful in fine-tuning and increasing the validity of the interview guide.

Focus Groups

Finally, focus groups were used to check or verify information collected from interviews and/or participant observation (see Scrimshaw and Hurtado 1987). Morgan (1988) suggests that focus groups provide access to information not easily obtained by either interviews or participant observation. First, unlike participant observation, focus groups allow for the observation of a significant amount of interaction on a topic in a limited amount of time. Second, unlike individual interviews, focus groups allow for group interaction. Just as with other methods, focus groups should not be the only source of data collection for qualitative research, but focus groups do add a tool to the "tool box" for uncovering insider meanings.

Focus groups may follow other methods or may be used to gather preliminary information when participant observation is not possible. However, the researcher should be aware of two major limitations: (1) the setting is unnatural, and (2) groups may be reluctant to discuss private or taboo topics and behaviors (Scrimshaw and Hurtado 1987).

The second limitation was particularly relevant for this project as the behaviors under study were sexual behaviors. In dealing with taboo topics, focus groups may create a consensus when in reality there is no consensus. Just as in interviews where the interviewee may tell the interviewer what he or she wants to hear, in focus groups the individual may go along with the group even though he or she feels differently, particularly if there are one or more strong personalities in the group. Therefore, in this project, questions regarding sexual behaviors discussed in the group were written on index cards. Participants were handed the cards with ink pens at the end of the focus group. The behaviors were written in statement form and participants were asked if they had participated in the behavior within a given period of time.

Appendix B

The Sample

Interview Sample

In the interview sample (*N*=30), twenty-eight (93 percent) were Caucasian and two (7 percent) were Latino. The mean income was $26,710. All the men were gay, HIV negative, and fell between the ages of thirty and forty-four. However, only four participants were over thirty-eight years old. The modal age range was thirty-three to thirty-five, with ten individuals falling within this range. This skewing of age to the lower end of the scale may have resulted because there are few men in West Hollywood who are both over thirty-eight years old and HIV negative.

The focus groups were similarly constituted. All thirteen focus group participants were Caucasian. Only two participants were over thirty-eight years of age, and the average income was $29,325

Procedure

The participants were not selected randomly. For the thirty interviews, flyers were placed in coffee houses, bars, and area shops in the gay enclave of West Hollywood, California, and at a local volunteer-based AIDS service organization. Participants were also recruited from one of the HIV prevention programs in which I was a participant observer. The flyer did not mention relapse but instead promoted the interviews as part of a study on gay sexuality.

The thirteen participants for the focus groups were selected in a similar fashion, using the same flyer, except they were not recruited from prevention programs or AIDS service organizations. For both focus groups and interviews, there was some degree of snowball sampling. Participants were asked to mention the study to friends and have them call for screening. To participate, the person had to meet four criteria; he had to be a (1) gay-identified male, (2) between the ages of thirty and forty-four, (3) with HIV-negative status, (4) who resided in or identified with the West Hollywood community.

Each interview participant was paid twenty-five dollars for the interview and each focus group participant received fifteen dollars at the session's end.

Interview Sample Results

As demonstrated in table 1, the most often cited sexual activities by interviewees were oral receptive and oral insertive sex, followed closely by anal insertive and anal receptive sex. Nonpenetrative acts such as mutual masturbation were less popular.

TABLE 1

Preferred Sexual Activity

Type of Pleasure	Number Reporting	Percent
Oral Receptive	21	70%
Oral Insertive	18	60%
Anal Receptive	16	53%
Anal Insertive	14	47%
Mutual Masturbation	6	20%

Based upon their reports, this emphasis on oral sex seemed to be because they viewed oral sex without a condom as a risk-reduction strategy in which penetration could still occur. None of the men reported using condoms for oral sex. They found using condoms for oral sex to be cumbersome and less pleasurable. This was confirmed in the focus groups. On the other hand, all reported other risk-reduction strategies when having oral sex. They seemed to be cautious about having open cuts and sores in their mouths. In addition, they reported strategies such as "pulling out" before ejaculation and not swallowing sperm if ejaculation occurred.

These men appeared to prefer oral sex since it allows for some type of penetration and is a lower-risk activity compared to anal sex without a condom. In addition, they found nonuse of condoms to be more gratifying not only in a physical way but also in an emotional way.

Similar reasons were given for the desire to have anal sex. However, in contrast to oral sex, all reported that they usually use condoms for anal sex. At the same time, twenty-three reported at least one anal sex encounter without a condom in the last year, and five reported having had an unsafe sex encounter in the last two to three years. The type of unsafe anal sex reported is presented in table 2.

This table shows that 86 percent of the men have experienced anal sex without a condom even though they reported that they knew it was risky, and half the sample had an anal-*receptive* experience without a condom. This is the highest-risk sexual activity for gay men.

Nonetheless, regardless if the act was insertive or receptive, nineteen of the thirty individuals interviewed said that anal sex without a condom felt better. Table 3 represents situational or emotional difference(s) which may have preceded the unsafe sexual event.

TABLE 2

Type of Anal Sex (*N*=30)

Type of Activity	Number Reporting	Percent
Anal Receptive	15	50%
Anal Insertive	11	36%
Both anal receptive and anal insertive	2	7%
Not available	2	7%

TABLE 3

Unsafe Differences (*N*=30)

Unsafe Difference	Number Reporting	Percent
Turned on by partner	23	77%
Heavy foreplay	10	53%
Alcohol use	7	23%
Other drugs	4	17%
In love	4	13%
Half-asleep	2	7%
Condom broke / Not available	2	7%
Other	3	10%

Four men reported that the unsafe partner was a lover (meaning significant other). Others met their sexual partners at a gym, bar, through a friend, or at a "cruise spot" such as a parking lot where men can meet sexual partners. For some (eighteen), the unsafe sex encounter was the first or second encounter with the partner and he may not have seen the partner again. Six of the men had dated the partner for a short period of time.

Some (twelve) thought that their partner was HIV negative while others (thirteen) were unsure. One person knew his partner was HIV infected and two did not share this information.

Seven of the men reported alcohol use. However, only two reported that they were intoxicated. One of these two also reported that his partner was extremely attractive and that he was sexually excited by him. In addition, three of the other five also reported heavy foreplay along with "light" alcohol use (one or two drinks). Further, two of the seven also reported marijuana use along with alcohol. Two other men reported the use of other drugs without the use of alcohol. One drug was cocaine and the other was ecstasy, a popular "designer" drug.

The four who reported "being in love" as a reason for unsafe sex are in relationships, although it may not be a monogamous one. These men reported that noncondom use was more pleasurable and that it signified trust. Both he and his partner probably tested HIV negative and took the test together.

The two men who reported that they were "half-asleep" had unsafe sex in the early morning hours, and it was initiated by the partner. For both men, when they woke up and were "able to think clearly," they stopped the encounter. Most had condoms available. Only one person reported that a condom was not available and that he chose to have unsafe anal sex. One man reported that the condom broke during intercourse, but it "felt so good that I couldn't stop."

Limitations

The sample size is small, so of course generalizations are uncertain. However, I have suggested throughout that the fuzzy experience of the individual may not be captured by huge studies based upon a large number of individuals. Interview data were not collected from the sexual partner, perhaps giving a one-sided view of the sexual encounter. This is problematic of my and many other studies, given the nature of the subject. Finally, data are retrospective and rely upon participant recall. Prospective studies using diaries may provide further, more valid data regarding these experiences. Such research could be incorporated into an intervention (see Gold 1995).

Bibliography

AIDS Project Los Angeles. 1995. *SexVibe*: issues for Spring 1995, July 1995, and August-September 1995.

Abramson, P. and S. Pinkerton, eds. 1995. *Sexual Nature, Sexual Culture*. Chicago: University of Chicago Press.

Ackerman, Diane. 1994. *A Natural History of Love*. New York: Random House.

———. 1990. *A Natural History of the Senses*. New York: Random House.

Adib, S. M. and J. G. Joseph et al. 1991. "Predictors of Relapse in Sexual Practices Among Homosexual Men." *AIDS Education and Prevention* 3: 293–304.

Ajzen, I. 1988. *Attitudes, Personality, and Behavior*. Milton Keynes, UK: Open University Press.

Albert, E. 1986. "Illness and Deviance: The Response of the Press to AIDS." In D. Feldman and T. Johnson, eds., *The Social Dimensions of AIDS: Method and Theory*, 163–78. New York: Praeger.

Altman, D. 1986. *AIDS in the Mind of America*. New York: Doubleday Anchor.

Bailey, R. and R. Aunger. 1995. "Sexuality, Infertility, and Sexually Transmitted Disease Among Farmers and Foragers in Central Africa." In Abramson and Pinkerton, eds., *Sexual Nature, Sexual Culture*, 195–222.

Bandura, Albert. 1989. "Perceived Self-efficacy in the Exercise of Control Over AIDS Infection." In V. M. Mays, G. W. Albee, and S. F. Schneider, eds., *Primary Prevention of AIDS: Psychological Approaches*, 128–41. Newbury Park, Calif.: Sage.

——. 1986. *Social Learning Theory*. Englewood Cliffs, N.J.: Prentice-Hall.

——. 1977. "Self-Efficacy: Toward a Unifying Theory of Behavioral Change." *Psychological Review* 84: 191–215.

Barre-Sinoussi, F. et al. 1983. "Isolation of a T-lymphotropic Retrovirus from a Patient at Risk for Acquired Immune Deficiency Syndrome." *Science* 220: 868–71.

Bauman, L. and E. Adair. 1992. "The Use of Ethnographic Interviewing to Inform Questionnaire Construction." *Health Education Quarterly* 19 (1): 9–24.

Bayer, R. 1989. *Private Acts, Social Consequences: AIDS and the Politics of Public Health*. New York: Free Press.

Becker, M. H. and J. G. Joseph. 1988. "AIDS and Behavioral Change to Reduce Risk: A Review." *American Journal of Public Health* 78 (7): 394–410.

Biddle, W. 1995. *A Field Guide to Germs*. New York: Henry Holt.

Bloor, M. J., N. P. McKeganey, A. Finlay, and M. A. Barnard. 1992. "The Inappropriateness of Psycho-Social Models of Risk Behaviour for Understanding HIV-Related Risk Practices Among Glasgow Male Prostitutes." *AIDS Care* 4 (1): 131–37.

Bolton, R. 1992. "Mapping Terra Incognita: Sex Research for AIDS Prevention—An Urgent Agenda for the 1990s." In G. Herdt and S. Lindenbaum, eds., *The Time of AIDS: Social Analysis, Theory, and Method*, 124–58.

Bolton, R., J. Vincke, R. Mak, and E. Dennehey. 1992. "Alcohol and Risky Sex: In Search of an Elusive Connection." *Medical Anthropology* 14: 323–63.

Bosga, M. and J. B. F. de Wit et al. 1995. "Differences in Perception of Risk for HIV Infection with Steady and Non-steady Partners Among Homosexual Men." *AIDS Education and Prevention* 7 (2): 103–15.

Briggs, C. L. "Native Metacommunicative Competence and the Incompetence of Fieldworkers." *Language and Society* 13: 1–28.

Brownell, K. D., G. A. Marlatt, E. Lichtenstein, and G. T. Wilson. 1986. "Understanding and Preventing Relapse." *American Psychologist* 41: 764–82.

Browning, G. 1994. *The Culture of Desire: Paradox and Perversity in the Lives of Gay Men*. New York: Vintage.

Bull, C. and J. Gallagher. 1994. "The Lost Generation." *The Advocate* 656 (May 31): 36–44.

Bullough, V. L. 1994. *Science in the Bedroom: The History of Sex Research*. New York: HarperCollins.

Cain, Roy. 1991. "Stigma Management and Gay Identity Development." *Social Work* 36 (1): 67–73.

Carrier, J. M. 1980. "Homosexual Behavior in Cross-cultural Perspective." In J. Marmor, ed., *Homosexual Behavior: A Modern Appraisal*, 100–22. New York: Basic Books.

———. 1977. "Sex-role Preference as an Explanatory Variable in Homosexual Behavior." *Archives of Sexual Behavior* 6 (1): 53–65.

Cass, V. 1979. "Homosexual Identity Formation: A Theoretical Model." *Journal of Homosexuality* 4 (3): 219–25.

Chmiel, J. S. and R. Detels et al. 1987. "Factors Associated with Prevalent Human Immunodeficiency Virus (HIV) Infection in the Multicenter AIDS Cohort Study." *American Journal of Epidemiology* 126 (4): 310–18.

Chng, L. C. and A. Moore. 1993. "Dangerous Liaison: A Study of HIV Risk Behavior Relapse among Gay Men." Paper presented at the annual meeting of the American Public Health Association, October 24–28, San Francisco.

City of West Hollywood, California. 1995 (September), *City News: A Publication of the City of West Hollywood.*

Clay, S. B. 1993. "Unsafe Sex Among Black Gay Men on the Rise." *HIV Educator* 1: 1 (published by the California AIDS Clearing House).

Coveney, P. and R. Highfield. 1995. *Frontiers of Complexity: The Search for Order in a Chaotic World.* New York: Fawcett Columbine.

Coyle, S., R. F. Boruch, and C. F. Turner. 1991. *Evaluating AIDS Prevention Programs.* Washington, D.C.: National Academy Press.

Cronin, H. 1991. *The Ant and the Peacock.* Cambridge: Cambridge University Press.

Cytowic, Richard. 1993. *The Man Who Tasted Shapes.* New York: Tarcher/ Putnam.

Daniel, H. and R. Parker. 1993. *Sexuality, Politics, and AIDS in Brazil: Another World?* London: Falmer Press.

Darwin, Charles. 1968 (originally published in 1859). *On the Origin of Species by Natural Selection.* London: Penguin.

Davies, P. M., F. C. I. Hickson, P. Weatherburn, and A. J. Hunt. 1993. *Sex, Gay Men, and AIDS.* London: Falmer Press.

Davis, M. S. 1983. *Smut: Erotic Reality/Obscene Ideology.* Chicago: University of Chicago Press.

Dawes, R. M. 1994. *House of Cards: Psychology and Psychotherapy Built on Myth.* New York: Free Press.

Dawkins, R. 1989. *The Selfish Gene.* Oxford and New York: Oxford University Press.

de Wit, J. B. F. and G. J. P. Van Griensven et al. 1993. "Why Do Homosexual Men Relapse into Unsafe Sex? Predictors of Resumption of Unprotected Anogenital Intercourse with Casual Partners." *AIDS* 7: 1113–18.

de Wit, J. B. F. and J. A. R. Van Den Hock et al. 1993. "Increase in Unprotected Anogenital Intercourse Among Homosexual Men." *American Journal of Public Health* 83 (10): 1451–53.

Díaz, R. and B. Marín. 1993. "Barriers to Safer Sex Practices Among Latino Gay Men in the USA." Paper presented at the annual meeting of the American Public Health Association, October 24–28, San Francisco.

Donovan, C., C. Mearns, R. McEwan, and N. Sugden. 1995. "A Review of the HIV-Related Sexual Behaviour of Gay Men and Men Who Have Sex with Men." *AIDS Care* 6 (5): 605–17.

Douglas, Mary. 1966. *Purity and Danger: An Analysis of the Concepts of Pollution and Taboo*. New York: Routledge and Kegan Paul.

Drlica, K. A. 1994. *Double-Edged Sword: The Promises and Risks of the Genetic Revolution*. Menlo Park, Calif.: Addison-Wesley.

Edgerton, Robert B. 1992. *Sick Societies: Challenging the Myth of Primitive Harmony*. New York: Free Press.

Ekstrand, M. L. 1992. "Safer Sex Maintenance Among Gay Men: Are We Making Any Progress?" *AIDS* 6: 875–77.

Ekstrand, M. L. and R. Stall. 1993. "Safer Sex Among Gay Men: What Is the Ultimate Good?" *AIDS* 7: 281–82.

Ekstrand, M. L. and T. J. Coates. 1990. "Maintenance of Safer Sexual Behaviors and Predictors of Risky Sex: The San Francisco Men's Health Study." *American Journal of Public Health* 80 (8): 973–77.

Ewald, Paul. 1994. *Evolution of Infectious Disease*. Oxford and New York: Oxford University Press.

Ewing, Katherine. 1990. "The Illusion of Wholeness: Culture, Self, and the Experience of Inconsistency." *Ethos* 18 (3): 251–78.

Foucault, Michel. 1978. *The History of Sexuality*, vol. 1, *An Introduction*. New York: Random House.

Frutchey, C. 1993. "Strategies for Maintaining Behavior Change." *HIV Educator* 1: 12–14 (published by the California AIDS Clearing House).

Furin, J. 1995. "Becoming My Own Doctor: Gay Men, AIDS, and Alternative Therapy Use in West Hollywood, California." Ph.D. diss. (anthropology), University of California at Los Angeles.

Gallo, Robert et al. 1984. "Frequent Detection and Isolation of Cytopathic Retroviruses (HTLV-III) from Patients with AIDS and at Risk for AIDS." *Science* 224: 500–503.

Garrett, L. 1994. *The Coming Plague: Newly Emerging Diseases in a World Out of Balance*. New York: Farrar, Straus, and Giroux.

Gatter, P. 1995. "Anthropology, HIV, and Contingent Identities." *Social Science and Medicine* 41 (11): 1523–33.

Gell-Mann, Murray. 1994. *The Quark and the Jaguar: Adventures in the Simple and the Complex*. New York: W. H. Freeman.

Glaser, B. G. and A. L. Strauss. 1967. *The Discovery of Grounded Theory: Strategies for Qualitative Research*. Chicago: Aldine.

Gold, R. 1995. "Why We Need to Rethink AIDS Education for Gay Men." *AIDS Care* 7 (1): S11–S19.

———. 1993. "On the Need to Mind the Gap: On-Line Versus Off-Line Cognitions Underlying Sexual Risk-Taking." In D. J. Terry, C. Gallois, and M. McCamish, eds., *The Theory of Reasoned Action: Its Application to AIDS-Preventive Behaviour*, 227–52. Oxford: Pergamon.

Gold, R., M. J. Skinner, P. J. Gront, and O.C. Plummer. 1991. "Situational Factors and Thought Processes Associated with Unprotected Intercourse in Gay Men." *Psychology and Health* 5 (4): 259–78.

Gorman, E. Michael. 1992. "The Pursuit of the Wish: An Anthropological Perspective on Gay Male Subculture in Los Angeles." In G. Herdt, ed., *Gay Culture in America*, 87–105. Boston: Beacon Press.

———. 1991. "Anthropological Reflections on the HIV Epidemic Among Gay Men." *Journal of Sex Research* 28 (2): 263–73.

Green, R. 1987. *The "Sissy-Boy Syndrome" and the Development of Homosexuality*. New Haven: Yale University Press.

———. 1985. "Gender Identity in Childhood and Later Sexual Orientation: Follow-up of Seventy-eight Males." *American Journal of Psychiatry* 142: 339–41, 142.

Greenberg, D. F. 1995. "The Pleasures of Homosexuality." In Abramson and Pinkerton, eds., *Sexual Nature, Sexual Culture*, 223–56.

———. 1988. *The Construction of Homosexuality*. Chicago: University of Chicago Press.

Gunn, Thom. 1989. "The Missing." In M. Klein, ed., *Poets for Life*, 986. New York: Crown.

Halstead, Fred. 1979. "An Interview with Fred Halstead." In Rosa von Praunheim, ed., *Army of Lovers*, 90–96. San Francisco: Gay Sunshine Press.

Hamer, Dean and Peter Copeland. 1994. *The Science of Desire: The Search for the Gay Gene and the Biology of Behavior*. New York: Simon and Schuster.

Harris, M. 1979. *Cultural Materialism: The Struggle for a Science of Culture*. New York: Random House.

Hart, G. and M. Boulton et al. 1992. "Relapse to Unsafe Sexual Behaviour Among Gay Men: A Critique of Recent Behavioural HIV/AIDS Research." *Sociology of Health and Illness* 14 (2): 217–31.

Harteis, Richard. 1989. "The Dolphins." In M. Klein, ed., *Poets for Life*, 996. New York: Crown.

Henrickson, M. 1994. "The Irony's in the Fire: Towards a Gay Epistemology." Comprehensive paper submitted in partial fulfillment of Ph.D. degree, University of California, Los Angeles.

Herdt, G. 1989. "Introduction: Gay and Lesbian Youth, Emergent Identities, and Cultural Scenes at Home and Abroad." *Journal of Homosexuality* 17 (1): 1–42.

——. 1987. *The Sambia: Ritual and Gender in New Guinea.* New York: Holt, Rinehart, and Winston.

Herdt, G., ed. 1992. *Gay Culture in America: Essays from the Field.* Boston: Beacon Press.

——, ed. 1984. *Ritualized Homosexuality in New Guinea.* Berkeley: University of California Press.

Herdt, G. and A. Boxer. 1991. "Ethnographic Issues in the Study of AIDS." *Journal of Sex Research* 28 (2): 171–87.

Herdt, G. and S. Lindenbaum, eds. 1992. *The Time of AIDS: Social Analysis, Theory, and Method.* Newbury Park, Calif.: Sage.

Herrel, R. 1992. "The Symbolic Strategies of Chicago's Gay and Lesbian Pride Day Parade." In G. Herdt, ed., *Gay Culture in America*, 225–52. Boston: Beacon Press.

Hobson, J. A. 1994. *The Chemistry of Conscious States: How the Brain Changes Its Mind.* Boston: Little, Brown.

Hospers, H. J. and G. Kok. 1995. "Determinants of Safe and Risk-taking Sexual Behavior Among Gay Men: A Review." *AIDS Education and Prevention* 7 (1): 74–94.

Hovland, C. I., I. L. Janis, and H. H. Kelley. 1953. *Communication and Persuasion.* New Haven: Yale University Press.

Joseph, J. G. and S. B. Montgomery et al. 1987a. "Magnitude and Determinants of Behavioral Risk Reduction: Longitudinal Analysis of a Cohort at Risk for AIDS." *Psychology and Health* 1: 73–95.

——. 1987b. "Perceived Risk of AIDS: Assessing the Behavioral Consequences in a Cohort of Gay Men." *Journal of Applied Social Psychology* 17: 231–50.

Jung, Carl. 1964. *Man and His Symbols.* New York: Dell.

Kanfer, F. H. 1980. "Self-Management Methods." In F. H. Kanfer and A. P. Goldstein, eds., *Helping People Change: A Textbook of Methods.* Elmsford, N.Y.: Pergamon.

——. 1971. "The Maintenance of Behavior by Self-generated Stimuli and Reinforcement." In A. Jacobs and L. B. Sachs, eds., *The Psychology of Private Events.* New York: Academy Press.

——. 1970. "Self-Regulation: Research, Issues, and Speculations." In C. Nueringer and J. L. Michael, eds., *Behavior Modification in Clinical Psychology.* New York; Appleton-Century-Crofts.

Kanouse, D. E., S. H. Berry, E. M. Gorman, E. M. Yano, and S. Carson. 1991. *Response to the AIDS Epidemic: A Survey of Homosexual and Bisexual Men in Los Angeles County.* Los Angeles: Rand.

Kaplan, H. S. 1979. *Disorders of Sexual Desire.* New York: Simon and Schuster.

Kelly, J. A. 1995. *Changing HIV Risk Behavior: Practical Strategies.* New York: Guilford Press.

Kelly, J. A. and J. S. St. Lawrence et al. 1990a. "AIDS Risk Behavior Among Gay Men in Small Southern Cities." *American Journal of Public Health* 80 (8): 416–18.

Kelly, J. A., J. S. St. Lawrence, T. L. Brasfield, A. L. Lemke, T. Amide, R. A. Roffman, H. V. Hood, J. E. Smith, H. Kilgore, and C. McNeill. 1990b. "Psychological Factors That Predict AIDS High-risk Versus AIDS Precautionary Behavior." *Journal of Consulting and Clinical Psychology* 58 (1): 117–20.

Kelly, J. A., J. S. St. Lawrence, H. V. Hood, and T. L. Brasfield. 1989. "Behavioral Interventions to Reduce AIDS Risk Activities." *Journal of Consulting and Clinical Psychology* 57 (1): 60–67.

Kelly J. A., J. S. St. Lawrence, and T. L. Brasfield. 1991. "Predictors of Vulnerability to AIDS Risk Behavior Relapse." *Journal of Consulting and Clinical Psychology* 59 (1): 163–66.

Kelly, J. A. and S. C. Kalichman et al. 1991. "Situational Factors Associated with AIDS Risk Behavior Lapses and Coping Strategies Used by Gay Men Who Successfully Avoid Lapses." *American Journal of Public Health* 81 (10): 1335–38.

Kennedy, M. P. 1992. "Preventing Relapse." *HIV Educator* 1: 15–19 (published by the California AIDS Clearing House.

Kippax, S. and J. Crawford et al. 1993. "Sustaining Safe Sex: A Longitudinal Study of a Sample of Homosexual Men." *AIDS* 7: 257–63.

Kirk, J. and M. L. Miller. 1988. *Reliability and Validity in Qualitative Research,* vol. 1 of *Qualitative Research Methods.* Newbury Park, Calif.: Sage.

Kosko, B. 1993. *Fuzzy Thinking: The New Science of Fuzzy Logic.* New York: Hyperion.

Koswicz, J. and T. Miller. 1993. "Perceptions of and Experiences with the Gay Community and Their Import for Gay Men in Maintaining Safer Sexual Behavior." Paper presented at the annual meeting of the American Public Health Association, October 24–28, San Francisco.

Kramer, Larry. 1989. *Reports from the Holocaust: The Making of an AIDS Activist.* New York: St. Martin's.

Lamptey, P. and T. Coates et al. 1993. "Prevention: Is it Working?" Plenary session at the Ninth Annual International Conference on AIDS, Berlin (PS-02–2).

Langness, L. L. 1965. *The Life History in Anthropological Science.* New York: Holt, Rinehart, and Winston.

Lappé, Marc. 1995. *Break Out: The Evolving Threat of Drug-resistant Disease.* San Francisco: Sierra Club.

LeVay, Simon. 1994. *The Sexual Brain.* Cambridge, Mass.: MIT Press.

Leventhal, H., O. Meyer, and M. Gutmann. 1980. "The Role of Theory in the Study of Compliance to High Blood Pressure Regimens." In R. B. Haynes, M. E. Mattson, and O. E. Tillmer, eds., *Patient Compliance to Prescribed Antihypertensive Medication Regimens: A Report to the National Heart, Lung, and Blood Institute.* Washington, D.C.: U.S. Department of Health and Human Services.

Levine, M. P. and K. Siegel. 1992. "Unprotected Sex: Understanding Gay Men's Participation." In J. Huber and B. E. Sneider, eds., *The Social Context of AIDS,* 139–57. Newbury Park, Calif.: Sage.

Levinton, L. C. 1989. "Theoretical Foundations of AIDS-Prevention Programs." In R. O. Valdiserri, ed., *Preventing AIDS: The Design of Effective Programs.* New Brunswick: Rutgers University Press.

Lewis, C. S. 1955. *The Magician's Nephew.* New York: Macmillan.

Liebowitz, M. 1983. *The Chemistry of Love.* Boston: Little, Brown.

Lyon, Judith. 1993. "Relational Power Schemas: Effects on Safer Sex." Ph.D. diss., University of California at Santa Barbara.

Malinowski, B. 1961 (originally published in 1922). *Argonauts of the Western Pacific.* New York: Dutton.

Marlatt, G. A. and J. R. Gordon. 1985. *Relapse Prevention: Maintenance Strategies in the Treatment of Addictive Behaviors.* New York: Guilford Press.

Martin, J. L. 1986. "AIDS Risk-Reduction Recommendations and Sexual Behavior Patterns Among Gay Men: A Multifactorial Categorical Approach to Assessing Change." *Health Education Quarterly* 13 (4): 346–58.

Masters, W. H. and V. E. Johnson. 1966. *Human Sexual Response.* Boston: Little, Brown.

McCusker, J. et al. 1992. "Maintenance of Behavioral Change in a Cohort of Homosexual Active Men." *AIDS* 6: 861–68.

McCusker, J., J. Zapka, A. M. Stoddard, and K. H. Mayer. 1989. "Responses to the AIDS Epidemic Among Homosexually Active Men: Factors Associated with Preventive Behavior." *Patient Education and Counseling* 13: 15–30.

McKusick, L. and M. Conant et al. 1985. "The AIDS Epidemic: A Model for Developing Intervention Strategies for Reducing High-Risk Behavior in Gay Men." *Sexually Transmitted Diseases* 12: 229–34.

McKusick, L. and T. J. Coates et al. 1990. "Longitudinal Predictors of Reductions in Unprotected Anal Intercourse Among Gay Men in San Francisco:

The AIDS Behavioral Research Project." *American Journal of Public Health* 80 (8): 978–83.

McWhirter, D. and W. Mattison. 1984. *The Male Couple: How Relationships Develop*. Englewood Cliffs, N.J.: Prentice-Hall.

Meyer, G., J. Dearing, and M. Casey. 1995. "Applying Social Marketing and Diffusion Strategies to HIV Prevention Programs in San Francisco." *Social Marketing Quarterly* 2 (1): 3–5.

Meyer, I. and L. Dean. 1995. "Patterns of Sexual Behavior and Risk-Taking Among Young New York City Gay Men." *AIDS Education and Prevention* 7 (supplement): 13–23.

Meyer-Bahlberg, H. F. L. 1995. "Psychoneuroendocrinology and Sexual Pleasure: The Aspect of Sexual Orientation." In Abramson and Pinkerton, eds., *Sexual Nature, Sexual Culture*, 135–53.

Miller, R. L. 1995. "Assisting Gay Men to Maintain Safer Sex: An Evaluation of an AIDS Service Organization's Safer Sex Maintenance Program." *AIDS Education and Prevention* 7 (supplement): 48–63.

Morgan, D. L. 1988. *Focus Groups as Qualitative Research*, vol. 16 of *Qualitative Research Methods*. Newbury Park, Calif.: Sage.

Monette, Paul. 1990. *Afterlife*. New York: Crown.

Money, John. 1961. "Sex Hormones and Other Variables in Human Eroticism." In W. C. Young, ed., *Sex Internal Secretions*, vol. 2. Baltimore: Williams and Wilkins.

Morris, M., J. Zavisca, and L. Dean. 1995. "Social and Sexual Networks: Their Role in the Spread of HIV/AIDS Among Young Gay Men." *AIDS Education and Prevention* 7 (supplement): 24–35.

Mosley, T. 1994. "Ten Years in a Cardboard Box: Memoirs of an APLA Survivor." *Frontiers* 12: 20.

Mulry, G., S. Kalichman, and J. Kelly. 1994. "Substance Abuse and Unsafe Sex Among Gay Men: Global Versus Situational Use of Substances." *Journal of Sex Education and Therapy* 20 (3): 175–84.

Murray, S. O. 1992. "Components of Gay Community in San Francisco." In G. Herdt, ed., *Gay Culture in America*. Boston: Beacon Press.

Neese, R. M. and G. C. Williams. 1994. *Why We Get Sick: The New Science of Darwinian Medicine*. New York: Times Books.

Odets, Walt. 1995. *In the Shadow of the Epidemic: Being HIV-Negative in the Age of AIDS*. Durham, N.C.: Duke University Press.

Ostrow, D. and W. J. DiFranceisco et al. 1995. "A Case-Control Study of Human Immunodeficiency Virus Type 1 Seroconversion and Risk-related Behaviors in the Chicago MACS/CCS Cohort, 1984–1992." *American Journal of Epidemiology* 142 (8): 875–83.

Panem, S. 1988. *The AIDS Bureaucracy*. Cambridge: Harvard University Press.

Pelto, P. and G. Pelto. 1978. *Anthropological Research: The Structure of Inquiry*. New York: Cambridge University Press.

Phillips, K. A. and J. Paul et al. 1995. "Predictors of Repeat HIV Testing Among Gay and Bisexual Men." *AIDS* 9: 769–75.

Phillips, K. A. and T. J. Coates. 1995. "HIV Counseling and Testing: Research and Policy Issues." *AIDS Care* 7 (2): 115–22.

Plummer, K. 1978. *Sexual Stigma: An Interactionist Account*. London: Falmer Press.

Preston, Richard. 1994. *The Hot Zone*. New York: Random House.

Prieur, A. 1990. "Norwegian Gay Men: Reasons for Continued Practice of Unsafe Sex." *AIDS Education and Prevention* 2 (2): 109–15.

Restak, R. 1994. *Receptors*. New York: Bantam.

Rice, R. and C. Atkin, eds. 1989. *Public Communication Campaigns*. Newbury Park, Calif.: Sage.

Ridley, M. 1993. *The Red Queen*. New York and London: Viking.

Rosen, R. and A. K. Ashton. 1992. "Prosexual Drugs: Empirical Status of the New Aphrodisiacs." *Archives of Sexual Behavior* 22 (6): 521–43.

Ryan, W. 1971. *Blaming the Victim*. New York: Vintage.

San Francisco AIDS Foundation. 1990. *HIV-related Knowledge, Attitudes, and Behaviors Among San Francisco Gay Men: Results from the Fifth Population Study*. San Francisco: Communication Technologies.

Schmidt, G. 1983. "Motivationale Grundlagen Sexuellen Verhaltens." In H. Thomä, ed., *Psychologie der Motive*, vol. 2 of *Motivation and Emotion* in the *Enzyklopädie der Psychologie*. Göttingen: Verlag für Psychologie.

Schneider, A. and B. Tarshis. 1986. *Physiological Psychology*. New York: McGraw-Hill.

Schunk, D. H. and J. P. Carbonari. 1984. "Self-Efficacy Models." In J. D. Matarazzo and J. A. Herd et al., *Behavioral Health: A Handbook of Health Enhancement and Disease Prevention*. New York: Wiley.

Scrimshaw, Susan C. M. 1990. "Combining Quantitative and Qualitative Methods in the Study of Intra-household Resource Allocation." In B. Rogers and N. Schlossman, eds., *Intra-household Resource Allocation: Issues and Methods for Development Policy and Planning*, 86–98. New York: United Nations University Press.

Scrimshaw, S. and E. Hurtado. 1987. *Rapid Assessment Procedures for Nutrition and Primary Health Care*. Los Angeles: Regents of the University of California and the United Nations University.

Sedgewick, E. 1990. *Epistemology of the Closet*. Berkeley: University of California Press.

Seibt, A. C. and M. W. Ross et al. 1995. "Relationship Between Safe Sex and Acculturation into the Gay Subculture." *AIDS Care* 7 (1): S85–S88.

Seligmann, M. (presenter for NRC/ANS Coordinating Committee). 1993. "The Concorde Trial: First Results." Paper presented at the Ninth Annual International Conference on AIDS, Berlin (WS-B24–5).

Shilts, Randy. 1987. *And the Band Played On: Politics, People, and the AIDS Epidemic*. New York: St. Martin's.

Siegel, K., F. P. Mesagno, J. Y. Chen, and G. Christ. 1989. "Factors Distinguishing Homosexual Males Practicing Risky and Safer Sex." *Social Science and Medicine* 28 (6): 561–69.

Siegel, K. and L. J. Bauman et al. 1988. "Patterns of Change in Sexual Behavior Among Gay Men in New York City." *Archives of Sexual Behavior* 17 (6): 481–97.

Silven, David. 1993. "Behavioral Therapies and Relapse." *Focus: A Guide to AIDS Research and Counseling* 8 (2): 1–8.

Simmons, T. 1995. "The Glamorization of AIDS." *The Advocate* 695 (November 28): 29.

Small, Meredith F. 1992. "What's Love Got to Do with It? Sex Among Our Closest Relatives Is a Rather Open Affair." *Discover* (June): 46–51.

Spradley, J. 1980. *Participant Observation*. San Francisco: Holt, Rinehart, and Winston.

Stall, R. and M. L. Ekstrand et al. 1990. "Relapse from Safer Sex: The Next Challenge for AIDS Prevention Efforts." *Journal of Acquired Immune Deficiency Syndrome* 3 (12): 1181–87.

Stall R., T. J. Coates, and C. Hoff. 1988. "Behavioral Risk Reduction for HIV Infection Among Gay and Bisexual Men: A Review of Results from the United States." *American Psychologist* 43 (11): 878–85.

Steckler, A. and K. Mcleroy et al. 1992. "Toward Integrating Qualitative and Quantitative Methods." *Health Education Quarterly* 19 (1): 1–8.

St. Lawrence, J. S. et al. 1990. "Factors Which Predict Relapse for Gay Men." Poster presented at the Sixth Annual International Conference on AIDS, San Francisco.

Sutton, S. R. 1982. "Fear-Arousing Communications: A Critical Examination of Theory and Research." In J. R. Eiser, ed., *Social Psychology and Behavioral Medicine*. New York: Wiley.

Tedesco, L. and M. Keffer. 1991. "Social Cognitive Theory and Relapse Prevention: Reframing Patient Compliance." *Journal of Dental Education* 55 (9): 575–82.

Tighe, J. C. 1991. *HIV Counselor Perspective: Relapse*. San Francisco: UCSF AIDS Health Project.

Torey, E. F. 1972. *The Mind Game*. New York: Bantam.

Turner, D. C. 1995. "HIV, Body Image, and Sexuality." *AIDS Patient Care* 9 (5): 245–48.

———. 1994. "For the Sake of Male Pleasure: Gay Identity, HIV, Grief, and Risky Sex." Ph.D. diss. (anthropology), University of California at Los Angeles.

———. 1991. "You Can Only Lead If We Follow: Internal Struggles of an AIDS Activist Group." Master's thesis (anthropology), University of California at Los Angeles.

Tuzin, D. 1995. "Discourse, Intercourse, and the Excluded Middle: Anthropology and the Problem of Sexual Experience." In Abramson and Pinkerton, eds., *Sexual Nature, Sexual Culture*, 257–75.

Udry, J. R. 1988. "Biological Predispositions and Social Control in Adolescent Sexual Behavior." *American Sociological Review* 53: 709–22.

Valdiserri, R. O., ed. 1989. *Preventing AIDS: The Design of Effective Programs*. New Brunswick: Rutgers University Press.

Valdiserri, R. O. et al. 1990. "Preventing HIV Infection in Gay and Bisexual Men: Experimental Evaluation of Attitude Change from Two Risk-Reduction Interventions." *AIDS Education and Prevention* 2 (2): 95–108.

Valdiserri, R. O., D. Lyter, L. Levinton, C. N. Callahan, L. A. Kingsley, and C. R. Rinaldo. 1989. "AIDS Prevention in Homosexual and Bisexual Men: Results of a Randomized Trial Evaluating Two Risk-Reduction Interventions." *AIDS* 3: 21–26.

———. 1989. "Variables Influencing Condom Use in a Cohort of Gay and Bisexual Men." *American Journal of Public Health* 78 (7): 801–803.

Vance, C. 1984. *Pleasure and Danger: Exploring Female Sexuality*. New York: Routledge and Kegan Paul.

Vermund, S. H. 1995. "Casual Sex and HIV Transmission" (editorial). *American Journal of Public Health* 85 (11): 1488–89.

Watney, S. 1988. "AIDS, Moral Panic, Theory, and Homophobia." In P. Appleton and H. Homans, eds., *Social Aspects of AIDS*, 52–82. London and New York: Falmer Press.

Watson, D. 1992. *Psychology*. Pacific Grove, Calif.: Brooks, Cole.

Watson, D. L. and R. G. Tharp. 1989. *Self-directed Behavior: Self-Modification for Personal Adjustment*. Pacific Grove, Calif.: Brooks, Cole.

Weatherburn, P. and P. Hunt et al. 1993. "No Connection Between Alcohol Use and Unsafe Sex Among Gay and Bisexual Men." *AIDS* 7: 115–19.

Weinrich, J. D. and I. Grant et al. 1993. "On the Effects of Childhood Gender Nonconformity on Adult Genito-Erotic Role and AIDS Exposure." *Archives of Sexual Behavior* 21 (6): 559–85.

Williams, L. S. 1986. "AIDS Risk Reduction: A Community Health Education Intervention for Minority High-Risk Group Members." *Health Education Quarterly* 13 (4): 407–21.

Williams, Tennessee. 1985 (originally published in 1954). "Hard Candy." In *Tennessee Williams: Collected Stories*. New York: New Directions.

Zadeh, L. 1965. "Fuzzy Sets." In *Information and Control* 8: 338.

Index

Between Men ~

Between Women

Lesbian and Gay Studies

Lillian Faderman and Larry Gross, Editors

Don Paulson with Roger Simpson, *An Evening in the Garden of Allah: A Gay Cabaret in Seattle*

Judith Roof, *Come As You Are: Sexuality and Narrative*

Judith Roof, *A Lure of Knowledge: Lesbian Sexuality and Theory*

Claudia Schoppmann, *Days of Masquerade: Life Stories of Lesbians During the Third Reich*

Alan Sinfield, *The Wilde Century: Effeminacy, Oscar Wilde, and the Queer Moment*

Jane McIntosh Snyder, *Lesbian Desire in the Lyrics of Sappho*

Chris Straayer: *Deviant Eyes, Deviant Bodies: Sexual Re-Orientations in Film and Video*

Thomas Waugh, *Hard to Imagine: Gay Male Eroticism in Photography and Film from Their Beginnings to Stonewall*

Kath Weston, *Families We Choose: Lesbians, Gays, Kinship*

Kath Weston, *Render me, Gender Me: Lesbians Talk Sex, Class, Color, Nation, Studmuffins...*

Carter Wilson, *Hidden in the Blood: A Personal Investigation of AIDS in the Yucatán*

NORWEGIAN
SOCIETY